Multiple

OPHTHAL

D F P Larkin, MRCPI, FCOphth
Lecturer in Ophthalmology
University of Bristol
England

Wolfe Publishing Ltd

Copyright © Wolfe Publishing Ltd.
Printed in Great Britain by
BPCC Hazell Books
Aylesbury, Bucks, England
Member of BPCC Ltd.

ISBN 0 7234 1671 0

A CIP catalogue record for this book is available from the British Library.

For a full list of Wolfe Atlases, plus forthcoming titles and details of our
surgical, dental and veterinary Atlases, please write to Wolfe Publishing
Ltd, 2–16 Torrington Place, London WC1E 7LT, England.

CONTENTS

PREFACE

This book is a collection of multiple choice questions drawn from the ophthalmic basic and clinical sciences. The multiple choice format of question is predominant in the written parts of the examinations of the new College of Ophthalmologists in Britain, and this collection will be helpful to candidates preparing for these, and similar, examinations in ophthalmology.

The aims are twofold. First, to familiarise candidates with the MCQ format and scoring system used, particularly those doctors unfamiliar with this question method. Second, to identify to readers any areas of weakness in their knowledge: this is of more importance than imparting new factual knowledge.

I am grateful to many ophthalmologists, particularly in the Bristol Eye Hospital, for reading the questions; to Professor David Easty for encouraging me to publish the questions in the first instance; and to Anne Williams for typing large sections of the text.

INTRODUCTION

There are two different types of multiple choice question (MCQ) that have become widely used in undergraduate and post-graduate medical examinations. The format given here is that used in all the MCQ examination papers of the College of Ophthalmologists and most MCQ examinations throughout the world. In this format, the question consists of a stem and five responses, of which any number may be correct. The Candidates answer true, false or omit that part of the question, according to their knowledge. Correct answers receive one mark and a mark is lost for each incorrect selection. No mark is given if a part of a question is omitted. Accordingly, the range of possible scores for each question group is +5 to −5; an overall pass mark of 50% is usually used and therefore candidates must aim to score at least +2.5 on average for each question.

The other question format used, particularly in North America, is the 'single correct response' type. The stem question or statement is followed by five responses of which only one is correct, which the candidate must identify.

With this collection of questions I have tried to strike a balance between basic science and clinical ophthalmology. The book is arranged into subspecialty chapters, following the module examination format used by the College of Ophthalmologists (consisting of separate papers in basic science, optics & refraction, and clinical ophthalmology). Readers will obtain most benefit if they mimic, as much as possible, examination conditions. Reach a true/false/omit decision on all questions before consulting the answers. Furthermore, allocate no more than two minutes for each question.

Bad performance in MCQ examination papers is not always due to poor knowledge of the subject. The +/− marking system described above leads to pitfalls, in particular for those unfamiliar with the MCQ format. This book will be particularly helpful in this respect.

QUESTIONS

Embryology and anatomy

1. The following structures are mesodermal in origin:

A   the dilator muscle of the iris
B   the iris stroma
C   the ciliary muscle
D   the ciliary epithelium
E   levator palpebrae superioris

2. The following are situated in the dorsal midbrain:

A   nucleus of Cajal
B   nucleus of the posterior commissure
C   rostral interstitial nucleus of the medial longitudinal bundle
D   third cranial nerve nucleus
E   Edinger–Westphal nucleus

3. Extraocular muscles

A   have a sensory nerve supply
B   light and electron microscopic appearances are typical of striated muscles
C   lateral rectus is supplied in part by the lacrimal artery
D   inferior rectus is supplied in part by the infra-orbital artery
E   smallest muscle mass is in the lateral rectus muscle

4. Concerning the trigeminal nerve:

A   ophthalmic division contains no motor supply
B   maxillary division contains no motor supply
C   mandibular division contains no motor supply
D   maxillary division passes through the inferior orbital fissure
E   Gasserian ganglion contains cell bodies of all trigeminal motor and sensory axons

5. **The following pass through the foramen ovale:**

A   maxillary division of trigeminal nerve
B   mandibular division of trigeminal nerve
C   motor root of trigeminal nerve
D   middle meningeal artery
E   lesser petrosal nerve

6. **Concerning the lacrimal gland:**

A   it is exocrine
B   it contains contractile myoepithelial cells
C   it receives parasympathetic, but not sympathetic, supply
D   neurons responsible for lacrimal secretion synapse in the geniculate ganglion
E   the Vidian nerve contains postganglionic lacrimal neurons

7. **The cornea**

A   is thinner at the centre than at the periphery
B   has an average central thickness of 0.96 mm
C   hemidesmosomes connect basal epithelial cells to basement membrane
D   Bowman's layer is acellular
E   stroma constitutes 75% of normal corneal thickness

8. **The following statements about the optic nerve are true:**

A   growth is complete six months after birth
B   it develops in the optic cup
C   myelin of fibres originates from Schwann cells
D   the nerve head is normally free of myelin
E   it is covered by pia, arachnoid and dura

9. **Concerning the anterior visual pathway:**

A   the ratio of crossed to uncrossed fibres in the chiasm is 53:47
B   the ganglion cell axons that arise from the retina temporal to a vertical line through the optic disc do not cross in the chiasm
C   the lateral geniculate body is part of the superior colliculus
D   histologically, each lateral geniculate body is composed of white matter
E   an inferior relation of the lateral geniculate body is the posterior cerebral artery

10. **In the hypothalamo-pituitary complex:**

A   the hypothalamus is located within the wall of the fourth ventricle
B   oxytocin is synthesised in the posterior pituitary
C   ADH is synthesised in the posterior pituitary
D   TRH is synthesised in the anterior pituitary
E   prolactin is synthesised in the anterior pituitary

11. **Regarding the orbital floor:**

A   the zygomatic bone is a constituent
B   the palatine bone is a constituent
C   the maxillary bone is a constituent
D   the lesser wing of sphenoid is a constituent
E   the lacrimal bone contains the nasolacrimal canal

12. **The left trochlear nerve**

A   nucleus is located in the midbrain at the level of the superior colliculus
B   leaves the brainstem on its dorsal aspect
C   passes inferior to the petroclinoid ligament
D   supplies the left superior oblique
E   enters the muscle cone

13. **Regarding posterior segment embryology:**

A   the retinal pigment epithelium differentiates from the inner, invaginated layer of the optic cup
B   the foetal fissure initially runs from the anterior rim of the cup to the distal optic stalk
C   closure of the foetal fissure commences at the posterior end
D   the pigment epithelial cells of the retina are the first in the body to produce melanin
E   macular development does not begin until the fifth month of gestation

14. **The lens**

A   develops from endoderm
B   the nucleus formed earliest is the foetal nucleus
C   growth of lens fibres continues throughout life
D   is involved in coloboma secondary to sectoral hypoplasia of the ciliary body and zonules
E   may be infected by microorganisms during development

15. The following originate from neural crest cells:

A   corneal stroma
B   uveal melanocytes
C   optic nerve, axons and glia
D   orbital bones
E   lacrimal gland

16. Regarding posterior segment embryology:

A   vascularisation of the nasal retina is complete before that of the temporal retina
B   the hyaloid vascular system develops from mesoderm
C   the hyaloid vascular system disappears in the second trimester
D   in the developed eye, the primary vitreous remains as Cloquet's canal
E   in the developed eye, secondary vitreous comprises most of the bulk of the vitreous

Physiology

17. Saccadic eye movements

A   may be vertical
B   may be torsional
C   may occur during sleep
D   velocity can be voluntarily controlled
E   maximum velocity is 200 degrees/second

18. Structures involved in the control of saccadic eye movements include:

A   cerebellum
B   superior colliculus
C   temporal cortex
D   posterior commissure
E   medial longitudinal bundle

19. Pursuit eye movements

A   have a longer latency (initiation time) than saccades
B   to the left are controlled by the right hemisphere
C   to the left are controlled by the right hemicerebellum
D   are controlled by the parieto-occipital cortex
E   are abnormal in a medial longitudinal bundle lesion

20. Accommodation

A is initiated by sympathetic stimulation
B increases the anteroposterior diameter of the lens
C in a normal 20-year-old increases the dioptric power of the eye by at least 15 dioptres
D power may be measured by placing convex lenses in front of the eye
E of 1 dioptre is associated with 1 prism dioptre of accommodative convergence

21. Dark adaptation

A is more rapid in rods than cones
B causes the eye to become more sensitive to red than blue light
C may be abnormally slow in primary biliary cirrhosis
D from bright photopic illumination takes ten minutes to complete
E may be abnormal in Refsum's disease

22. The following statements about tear film are true:

A volume is approximately 30 μl
B protein content is 60% albumin
C immunoglobulin composition is 80% IgA
D lysozyme concentration is greater than in any other body fluid
E aqueous phase is deficient in vitamin A deficiency

23. The cornea

A obtains glucose mainly from the tear film and limbal capillaries
B endothelium obtains most of its oxygen from aqueous humour
C Descemet's membrane thickens with age
D swells only in the anteroposterior direction
E will not swell if excised and placed in a solution isotonic to plasma

24. Intraocular pressure

A varies ± 1 mmHg with phases of the arterial pulse
B varies ± 1 mmHg with phases of respiration
C is higher in early than in late morning
D decreases promptly at onset of sleep
E may be decreased by lowering blood osmolarity

25. **The following statements about vitreous humour are true:**

A volume in each globe is approximately 5.3 ml
B glucose content is important for retinal function
C viscosity is primarily due to collagen content
D water content is 89%
E absorbs some visible light

26. **The following statements about the lens are true:**

A water content is 66%
B protein content is 10%
C has a higher sodium content than aqueous humour
D has a higher potassium content than aqueous humour
E new fibres develop throughout life

27. **The following are abundant neurotransmitters in the human retina:**

A γ-aminobutyric acid
B adrenaline
C noradrenaline
D acetylcholine
E Substance P

28. **Vitamin A**

A is stored primarily in the retina
B is fat-soluble
C overdose can cause optic disc swelling
D milk is a poor dietary source
E deficiency can be caused by renal disease

29. **In the human retina:**

A rod density is maximal 3 mm from the fovea
B there are more cones than rods
C photoreceptors receive nutrition from the choroid
D horizontal cells are situated in the outer nuclear layer
E rods have no role in colour vision

30. **The following statements about the optic nerve are true:**

A   axonal transport is unidirectional
B   papilloedema does not occur in an eye with antecedent optic atrophy
C   macular fibres enter the nerve in a group on the nasal side
D   function in a patient with lens opacity can be usefully assessed by a pattern VER
E   115 msec is the upper limit of normal VER latency

31. **Concerning the electroretinogram:**

A   photoreceptors are responsible for the a-wave
B   bipolar cells are responsible for the b-wave
C   Müller cells are responsible for the c-wave
D   rod and cone components are separated on the basis of their spectral sensitivities
E   the a-wave is a positive deflection

32. **Aqueous humour**

A   is formed by ultrafiltration
B   is formed by active secretion
C   is formed by diffusion
D   differs from plasma in the virtual absence of protein
E   has the same content of vitamin C as plasma

Pathology

33. **Herpes viruses**

A   are RNA viruses
B   include varicella-zoster virus
C   include pox virus
D   include Epstein–Barr virus
E   include cytomegalovirus

34. **Langhans' giant cells are a feature of:**

A   juvenile xanthogranuloma
B   tuberculosis
C   foreign body reaction
D   chalazion
E   sarcoidosis

35. **The following types of cell function primarily in the initial phases of inflammation:**

A   eosinophils
B   basophils
C   T-lymphocytes
D   polymorphonuclear leucocytes
E   plasma cells

36. **Stains appropriate for diagnosis of fungal infection include**

A   haematoxylin and eosin
B   Giemsa
C   periodic acid-Schiff
D   Gomori methenamine silver
E   Ziehl–Neelsen

37. **The following organisms are Gram-negative:**

A   *Corynebacterium diphtheriae*
B   *Neisseria gonorrhoeae*
C   *Treponema pallidum*
D   *Streptococcus pneumoniae*
E   *Actinomyces israelii*

38. **Keratoacanthoma**

A   may be difficult to distinguish from a basal cell carcinoma on microscopy
B   is most common in young adults
C   is characterised by a dense infiltrate of lymphocytes
D   is typically crater-shaped
E   may spontaneously regress

39. **Squamous cell carcinoma of the eyelid**

A   is less common than basal cell carcinoma
B   rarely arises in normal skin
C   spreads to lymph nodes
D   prognosis is worse if there is formation of keratin pearls
E   is characterised by a dense inflammatory cell infiltrate

40. **Conjunctival intraepithelial neoplasia (carcinoma *in situ*) is characterised by**

A intact basement membrane of the epithelium
B spread to involve the corneal epithelium
C an avascular grey plaque
D low recurrence rate following excision biopsy
E rare transformation into invasive squamous carcinoma

41. **The following statements about corneal dystrophies are true:**

A they are always bilateral
B Bowman's layer is predominantly affected in Reis–Bückler's dystrophy
C Masson's trichrome stain is used in the diagnosis of macular dystrophy
D Congo Red stain is used in the diagnosis of lattice dystrophy
E deposition of glycosaminoglycan occurs in Fuchs' endothelial dystrophy

42. **Features of proliferative vitreoretinopathy include:**

A retinal pigment epithelium-derived cells in the vitreous
B exudative retinal detachment
C membrane formation on the posterior (subretinal) surface of the retina
D membrane formation on the posterior surface of detached vitreous
E good prognosis following surgical treatment

43. **In retinoblastoma:**

A calcification is an important diagnostic feature
B rosettes indicate a poorer prognosis
C a second non-ocular malignancy is more likely if the ocular tumour is unilateral
D haematogenous spread occurs more commonly than in uveal melanoma
E the extent of choroidal and optic nerve invasion have equal prognostic importance

44. **Uveal melanoma**

A   is commoner in black than in white patients
B   consisting of epithelioid cells contain giant cells
C   prognosis is worst for epithelioid cell type tumours
D   size is an important prognostic indicator
E   is most commonly of spindle A type

45. **Metastatic intraocular tumours**

A   usually arise from haematogenous spread via the central
      retinal artery
B   rarely rupture Bruch's membrane
C   commonly arise by local spread of an orbital neoplasm
D   are most commonly located at the macula
E   differ from choroidal melanomas in not causing serous
      retinal detachment

46. **Lacrimal gland tumours**

A   of benign mixed type are the most common
B   of benign mixed type are surrounded by a pseudocapsule
C   must not be biopsied if suspected to be of benign mixed cell
      type
D   of adenoid cystic type arise from ductal epithelium
E   of adenoid cystic type are characteristically painless

47. **Concerning secondary orbital tumours:**

A   they are more common than metastatic choroidal tumours
B   the maxillary sinus is the most common primary site
C   secondary orbital neuroblastoma usually occurs in the
      young adult age group
D   orbital neuroblastoma presents with proptosis
E   orbital neuroblastoma tends to invade orbital bones

48. **Features of primary open-angle glaucoma include:**

A   ganglion cell loss
B   photoreceptor loss
C   staphyloma
D   displacement of the lamina cribrosa
E   widening of pial septa in the optic nerve

49. You are asked to investigate conjunctival discharge in a 5-day-old infant. The following staining and culture methods are appropriate:

A   Giemsa stain
B   Gram stain
C   viral transport medium
D   Thayer–Martin medium
E   Löwenstein–Jensen medium

50. Optic nerve glioma

A   arises from the arachnoid within the dura
B   sections rarely contain mitotic figures or cellular atypia
C   typically causes a brisk leptomeningeal inflammation
D   characteristically presents with progressive visual loss but little proptosis
E   is usually seen in middle-aged females.

51. Corynebacteria

A   are Gram-positive cocci
B   are a constituent of the normal commensal population in the conjunctival sac
C   cause membranous conjunctivitis
D   are a recognised cause of phlyctenular conjunctivitis
E   are widely resistant to antibiotics

52. *Chlamydia trachomatis* serotype D causes

A   trachoma
B   non-specific urethritis
C   adult inclusion conjunctivitis
D   ophthalmia neonatorum
E   lymphogranuloma venereum

Pharmacology

53. The following inhibit bacterial cell wall synthesis:

A   chloramphenicol
B   tetracycline
C   aminoglycosides
D   penicillins
E   sulphonamides

54. The following adverse effects may be seen following long term oral corticosteroid therapy:

A proximal myopathy
B hyperglycaemia
C pancreatitis
D hyperkalaemia
E lymphocytopenia

55. Acetazolamide

A acts on the proximal convoluted tubule of the kidney
B effect on IOP correlates with diuretic action
C increases renal excretion of sodium
D may cause fatal metabolic alkalosis
E may cause cicatrising conjunctivitis

56. Acetylcholine

A acts at sympathetic autonomic ganglia
B acts at parasympathetic autonomic ganglia
C acts at most sympathetic peripheral nerve endings
D acts at most parasympathetic peripheral nerve endings
E is administered by intraocular injection

57. 30 minutes following instillation of a drop into the normal eye of an emmetropic 20-year-old, there is mydriasis, and the near point of accommodation is 10 cm.
The drop could be:

A phenylephrine
B guanethidine
C physostigmine
D cocaine
E cyclopentolate

58. Regarding transmission of nerve impulses:

A preganglionic autonomic neurons are myelinated
B postganglionic autonomic neurons are myelinated
C each parasympathetic, preganglionic neuron synapses with only one postganglionic neuron
D catechol-O-methyltransferase inactivates acetylcholine
E monoamine oxidase inactivates noradrenaline

59. **The following statements about antimicrobial agents are true:**

A   natamycin is an aminoglycoside
B   neomycin is an aminoglycoside
C   clindamycin is an aminoglycoside
D   amphotericin B is a polyene
E   ampicillin is a penicillinase-resistant penicillin

60. **The following statements about enzymes are true:**

A   cyclooxygenase converts leukotriene into arachidonic acid
B   aldose reductase converts glucose to sorbitol
C   aldose reductase converts galactose to dulcitol
D   tyrosinase converts DOPA to dopaquinone
E   galactose kinase converts galactose-1-phosphate to glucose-1-phosphate

61. **The following statements about neuromuscular transmission are true:**

A   pilocarpine is a nicotinic cholinergic agent
B   pilocarpine is used in the diagnosis of anisocoria
C   pilocarpine may induce hypermetropia
D   atropine is a muscarinic antagonist
E   botulinum toxin blocks neuromuscular transmission by reducing acetylcholine release from presynaptic terminals

62. **Ecothiopate (Phospholine Iodide)**

A   is a cholinesterase inhibitor
B   therapy may cause apnoea on succinylcholine administration
C   concomitant phenylephrine drops minimise production of iris cysts
D   causes cataract formation
E   is used in treatment of lice infestation of lashes

63. **Mannitol is**

A   contraindicated in heart failure
B   contraindicated in renal disease
C   never administered orally
D   given as a 2% solution
E   effective by draining water from aqueous and vitreous

64. **Intravenous gentamicin**

A   can cause vestibular toxicity
B   can cause auditory toxicity
C   is contraindicated in patients with renal impairment
D   is contraindicated in patients with myasthenia gravis
E   solution may be safely administered as an intravitreal injection

65. **Concerning antiviral agents:**

A   idoxuridine may be administered by drops and ointment
B   acyclovir (acycloguanosine) may be administered by drops and ointment
C   acyclovir is a purine derivative
D   acyclovir is activated only within virus-infected cells
E   viral resistance to acyclovir may lead to treatment failure

66. **The following drugs may cause benign intracranial hypertension:**

A   corticosteroids
B   acetazolamide
C   nalidixic acid
D   vitamin A
E   ethambutol

67. **Conjunctival scarring is a recognised adverse effect of treatment with**

A   'Ganda'
B   sulphamethoxazole
C   practolol
D   tetracycline
E   phenobarbitone

68. **Abnormal colour vision may be found in patients on treatment with:**

A   digitalis
B   chloroquine
C   gold
D   indomethacin
E   isoniazid

Statistics

69. **The following statements about standard deviation are true:**

A   standard deviation of a sample is the same as population standard deviation

B   standard deviation equals the square of the variance

C   95% of observations lie within one standard deviation of the mean

D   the standard deviation depends on the number of observations

E   the standard deviation always has a positive value

70. **The following statements are true:**

A   the larger the sample size, the greater the standard error

B   a value of $p < 0.01$ is less significant than $p > 0.01$

C   data which is non-parametric is assumed to be normally distributed

D   in a t-test, the null hypothesis is assumed in all cases

E   in a normal distribution, the mean, mode and median are equal in value

71. **In the chi-square test:**

A   the value of chi-square may be negative

B   the higher the chi-square value, the greater the significance

C   the null hypothesis is assumed in all cases

D   the difference between observed and expected frequencies is measured

E $p < 0.5$ is conventionally accepted as significant

Genetics

72. **An X-linked recessive condition**

A   is manifest in females only when the gene is in the homozygous state

B   is transmitted by affected males and by female carriers

C   all daughters of an affected male are carriers

D   all sons of an affected male are affected

E   if a female carrier marries a normal male, half of her sons will be affected

73. Autosomal dominant inheritance is seen in:

A homocystinuria
B Marfan's syndrome
C Fabry's disease
D dystrophia myotonica
E Best's macular dystrophy

74. X-linked inheritance is seen in:

A tritanopia
B deuteranomaly
C oculocutaneous albinism
D choroideraemia
E histiocytosis X

Optics

75. The image formed by a prism is:

A inverted
B virtual
C displaced away from the apex of the prism
D deviated by an angle which equals half the refractory angle of the prism
E deviated $1°$ by a prism of 1 prism dioptre power

76. In correction of esodeviation:

A base out prisms are used
B Fresnel prisms are suitable for longterm therapy
C decentration of spectacle lenses is not effective
D prism correction may be divided between the two eyes
E prisms are more suitable than surgery in most patients

77. Regarding a convex lens:

A light parallel to the principal axis is converged to the nodal point
B the principal axis intersects the principal plane at the nodal point
C a ray passing through the nodal point is undeviated
D a plus $(+)$ sign is appropriate
E the image of an object outside the focal length is erect and magnified

78. **Regarding a convex lens:**

A   lenses with a short focal length are more powerful than those with a long focal length

B   the prismatic effect is decreased towards the periphery of the lens

C   poor centration of lenses produces an unwanted prismatic effect

D   the prismatic effect is responsible for chromatic aberration

E   the prismatic effect is responsible for spherical aberration

79. **Regarding the Maddox rod:**

A   it consists of a series of spherical lenses

B   the patient views a white point source of light through it

C   the patient views a white line source of light through it

D   a line of light is seen perpendicular to the axis of the Maddox rod

E   the line image seen by the patient is white

80. **The following statements about cylindrical lenses are true:**

A   there is no vergence power in the axis of the cylinder

B   in the meridian at right angles to the axis, the cylinder acts as a spherical lens

C   the Jackson cross-cylinder is a cylindrical lens

D   the cross-cylinder is used to check the power of a cylinder

E   the cross-cylinder is used to check the axis of a cylinder

81. **Regarding aberrations:**

A   chromatic aberration is corrected by an aspheric lens

B   chromatic aberration is the basis of the duochrome test

C   in the duochrome test, a myopic eye sees the green letters more distinctly

D   the Stiles–Crawford effect reduces ocular spherical aberration

E   the impairment of visual acuity that occurs on wide mydriasis is due to spherical aberration

82.   **Regarding refraction by the eye:**

A   the far point in the emmetropic eye is at infinity
B   the near point of distant vision is the nearest point at which an object can be clearly seen when accommodation is not used
C   the amplitude of accommodation is the difference in dioptric power between the eye at rest and the fully accommodated eye
D   to focus an object at 25 cm, the emmetropic eye must exert 4 dioptres of accommodative power
E   in accommodation most of the change in lens curvature occurs at the posterior lens surface

83.   **Regarding ametropia:**

A   in ametropia the eye fails to bring parallel rays of light to a focus on the retina
B   in hypermetropia the far point is in front of the retina
C   in myopia the far point is between the eye and infinity
D   axial hypermetropia occurs when the eye is short relative to its focal power
E   aphakia is an example of axial hypermetropia

84.   **Regarding the human eye:**

A   all refractive errors are corrected to 6/6 with a pinhole diaphragm
B   the far point is in conjugate focus with the retina when the eye is not accommodated
C   in an uncorrected hypermetropic eye, the image falls behind the retina
D   spectacle correction in aphakia produces a relative spectacle magnification of 1.1
E   the ring scotoma perceived in aphakic correction is due to prismatic effect of spectacle lenses

85.   **Regarding the indirect ophthalmoscope:**

A   the field of view is largest in hypermetropia
B   condensing lenses are aspheric
C   the field of view is several times larger than that of the direct ophthalmoscope
D   the image of the patient's retina is virtual
E   the image of the patient's retina is erect

86. **The following statements about optical instruments are true:**

A   the neutral point of retinoscopy is reached when the patient's far point connects with the observer's nodal point

B   in retinoscopy at 0.66 m, the correction for working distance is 0.66D

C   direct ophthalmoscopy is more useful than indirect in patients with opacities of the ocular media

D   the keratometer measures the radius of curvature of the cornea

E   keratometry assesses only the central zone of the cornea

87. **Concerning optical instruments:**

A   the Hruby lens is convex

B   the Hruby lens dioptre power is 58.6D

C   the Hruby lens forms an inverted image of illuminated retina

D   the Hruby lens can be used without the slit lamp microscope

E   the area of contact of the Goldmann applanation tonometer is 3.06 mm in diameter

88. **Concerning the human eye:**

A   in a patient with axial myopia of −19D, emmetropia will result from lens extraction

B   a patient with 3D of myopia has a far point at 33 cm

C   in infancy, the eye is capable of greater than 25D of accommodation

D   a patient with 3D of hypermetropia needs to exert 0.33D of accommodation to see clearly at infinity

E   aniseikonia is a difference in retinal image size in the two eyes

89. **In the direct ophthalmoscope:**

A   the area of retina seen at one time is greater in a myopic than an emmetropic eye

B   the area of retina seen at one time depends on the distance between patient and observer

C   a convex lens is necessary in order to obtain a focussed image of the retina of a hypermetropic patient

D   the magnification is ×15 in an emmetropic eye

E   the area of retina seen at one time depends on the size of the pupil

90. **Light**

A   may be absorbed by the normal human lens
B   rays may be deviated by collagen fibres of the cornea
C   composed of waves exactly in phase is termed *polarised*
D   of one pure wavelength is termed *collimated*
E   diffraction is caused by the cornea

91. **The refractive index of the following exceed that of the cornea**

A   aqueous humour
B   crystalline lens cortex
C   crystalline lens nucleus
D   vitreous humour
E   crown glass

92. **Incident rays of light parallel to the principal axis**

A   are reflected towards the principal focus of a convex mirror
B   pass through the second principal focus of a convex lens
C   pass through the first principal focus of a concave lens
D   will converge to a point focus at a convex spherical curved surface if the refractive index of the second medium exceeds that of the first
E   of a cylindrical lens are converged

93. **In contact lens correction of myopia:**

A   the image is smaller than with spectacles
B   the field of vision is larger than with spectacles
C   less convergence is needed than with spectacles
D   more accommodation is needed than with spectacles
E   image size in refractive myopia is equalised

94. **Regarding soft contact lenses:**

A   the basic plastic is polymethylmethacrylate (PMMA)
B   thermal disinfection methods are contraindicated to avoid lens damage
C   hydrogen peroxide disinfection is suitable
D   they have little value in correction of astigmatism
E   they are contraindicated in a patient with a history of recurrent corneal erosion

95. **Contact lens wear results in**

A   decreased corneal sensation
B   corneal epithelial oedema
C   decreased availability of glucose for corneal metabolism
D   morphological endothelial cell changes
E   band keratopathy

96. **The following statements about laser are true:**

A   for a small spot size, it takes more energy per unit area to produce photocoagulation than with a large spot size
B   the wavelength of argon blue laser is 514 nm
C   argon green light is absorbed by melanin and xanthophyll pigments
D   krypton red laser is not absorbed by xanthophyll
E   more power is needed by longer wavelengths to achieve the same effect

Lids and lacrimal apparatus

97. **Entropion**

A   of the upper lid is always cicatricial
B   which is congenital only involves the lower lid
C   which is congenital requires treatment in most cases
D   which is involutional can be treated by lower lid retractor shortening
E   which is involutional can be treated by Zeigler cautery of skin

98. **Ectropion**

A   of the upper lid is most damaging to the cornea
B   of acute onset may be precipitated by intraocular surgery
C   is associated with blepharophimosis syndrome
D   is associated with dystrophia myotonica
E   is associated with leprosy

99. **Characteristic features of essential blepharospasm include:**

A   no interference with vision
B   unilaterality
C   associated dystonia of other facial muscles
D   persistence during sleep
E   good response to botulinum toxin A

100. **Characteristic features of blepharophimosis syndrome include:**

A   X-linked inheritance
B   distichiasis
C   telecanthus
D   ptosis
E   normal IQ

101. **In assessment of a patient with bilateral ptosis, the following features support a diagnosis of myasthenia gravis:**

A   asymmetrical involvement
B   ECG abnormalities
C   diplopia
D   normal pupils
E   family history of ptosis

102. **The Marcus Gunn jaw-winking phenomenon is**

A   a cause of ptosis which varies with movement of the jaw
B   due to synkinesis between levator palpebrae superioris and the facial muscles
C   treated by levator resection in some cases
D   always unilateral
E   always congenital

103. **The Fasanella–Servat operation**

A   is used in correction of ptosis in which levator function is 5–12 mm
B   is restricted to cases with ptosis of 1–2 mm
C   includes excision of part of Müller's muscle
D   is commonly complicated by conjunctival prolapse
E   is commonly complicated by corneal abrasion

104. **Concerning levator muscle resection:**

A   some levator function prior to surgery must always be present
B   large resections should be performed transconjunctivally rather than through the skin
C   with levator function of 5 mm, 15 mm of resection is appropriate
D   general anaesthesia is preferable to local anaesthesia
E   a Frost suture is placed in the upper lid margin at the end of surgery to protect the cornea for 48 hours

105. **Features more characteristic of seborrhoeic than staphylococcal marginal blepharitis include:**

A   loss of lashes
B   chalazion
C   inferior corneal punctate epitheliopathy
D   marginal keratitis
E   symptomatic response to topical prednisolone

106. **The following statements about malignant eyelid tumours are true:**

A   tumours within 10 mm of the lid margin require a full thickness excision
B   tumours fixed to the tarsal plate require a full thickness excision
C   basal cell carcinoma at the medial canthus are particularly suited to radiotherapy
D   sebaceous gland carcinoma arises only from the meibomian glands
E   squamous cell carcinoma accounts for 5% of malignant lid tumours

107. **Molluscum contagiosum**

A   is most common in young adults
B   is caused by infestation with lice
C   lesions are waxy nodules
D   may primarily involve the lid skin or conjunctiva
E   infected cells contain eosinophilic inclusion bodies

108. **A patient has epiphora. Syringe irrigation of the drainage system demonstrates patency. The following statements are true:**

A   *Actinomyces* canaliculitis typically causes this presentation
B   lacrimal sac tumours cause these findings
C   Jones dye tests are of value only if the drainage system can be successfully irrigated by syringe
D   if the Jones secondary irrigation test is negative, DCR will fail
E   successful syringe irrigation implies that hyper-lacrimation rather than drainage obstruction is the cause of epiphora

109. **The following lid tumours have malignant potential:**

A   basal cell papilloma
B   senile (solar) keratosis
C   keratoacanthoma
D   capillary haemangioma
E   neurofibroma

110. **Acquired causes of canalicular obstruction include**

A   weakness of the lacrimal pump
B   Herpes simplex infection
C   Stevens–Johnson syndrome
D   topical idoxuridine
E   nasal tumour

111. **You are asked to manage an elderly patient with acute dacryocystitis. The following statements are true:**

A   probing should be performed to confirm obstruction of the nasolacrimal duct
B   oral antibiotics are indicated
C   parenteral antibiotics are indicated
D   dacryocystorhinostomy should be performed on the next available operating list
E   acute ethmoid sinusitis is a possible differential diagnosis

Orbit

112. Dysthyroid eye disease

A is invariably associated with biochemical evidence of hyperthyroidism
B may be associated with psychiatric disturbance
C is the most common cause of non-axial proptosis
D is associated with erythema nodosum
E is associated with finger clubbing

113. Which of the following orbital diseases are more common in children than the elderly?

A metastatic neuroblastoma
B capillary haemangioma
C lymphoma
D secondary malignant neoplasms
E vasculitic lesions

114. Cavernous haemangioma

A is the most common primary orbital tumour
B presents as acute proptosis
C presents in childhood
D is usually situated outside the muscle cone
E is diagnosed by orbital venography

115. An orbital varix characteristically

A presents in childhood
B causes pulsatile proptosis
C causes visual loss
D resolves spontaneously
E responds to intralesional steroid injection

116. Features of caroticocavernous fistula include:

A bilateral clinical signs
B dilated superior ophthalmic vein on CT scan
C anterior segment ischaemia
D central retinal artery occlusion
E venous stasis retinopathy

117. **Features of idiopathic orbital pseudotumour include:**

A rapid onset
B presentation in the elderly in most cases
C spontaneous remission
D recurrence in the contralateral orbit
E response to systemic corticosteroid

118. **Orbital rhabdomyosarcoma**

A is the most common primary orbital malignant tumour in childhood
B usually causes medial displacement of the globe
C rarely necessitates exenteration
D biopsy may be harmful and should be avoided
E characteristically causes pain

119. **Blow-out fracture of the orbital floor**

A typically involves the orbital margin
B rarely causes damage to the globe
C gives a positive forced duction test
D causes pupil constriction in some cases
E causes enophthalmos more often than proptosis

120. **Benign mixed cell tumour of the lacrimal gland**

A tends to occur later in life than adenoid cystic carcinoma
B does not cause pain
C has a shorter history than adenoid cystic carcinoma
D has a bad prognosis
E should be biopsied through a lateral orbitotomy before a decision on treatment is made

121. **The following statements on orbital cellulitis are true:**

A ampicillin is an appropriate antibiotic
B cloxacillin is an appropriate antibiotic
C in a patient whose clinical status on intravenous antibiotics is unchanged, a subperiosteal abscess should be suspected
D in a patient whose clinical status on intravenous antibiotics is unchanged, cavernous sinus thrombosis should be suspected
E *Mucor* infection is usually seen in patients with systemic disease

122. **Capillary haemangioma**

A   first presents in adult life
B   when involving the skin, blanches on pressure
C   usually requires no treatment
D   is best treated initially with intralesional corticosteroid injection
E   is usually well encapsulated

123. **Concerning orbital surgery and trauma:**

A   lateral orbitotomy is indicated when a tumour is located within the muscle cone
B   lateral orbitotomy is particularly suitable for childhood orbital surgery
C   orbital decompression includes removal of the medial orbital wall
D   the orbit is not involved in a Le Fort III fracture
E   surgery is usually necessary for medial wall blow-out fracture

124. **Indications for surgery in blow-out fracture include:**

A   any diplopia persisting for two weeks
B   any radiologically demonstrated fracture in the orbital floor
C   enophthalmos greater than 2 mm
D   proptosis
E   infraorbital nerve involvement in the fracture

125. **In the management of dysthyroid eye disease:**

A   radiation therapy is effective in the management of proptosis
B   orbital decompression surgery usually diminishes strabismus
C   strabismus surgery is performed only in the presence of severe symptoms
D   strabismus surgery, as a rule, is preceded by trials with prisms
E   strabismus surgery causes proptosis to decrease

126. **Orbital cellulitis**

A   is most frequently caused by sinus infection
B   is associated with non-axial displacement of the globe
C   is usually accompanied by fever
D   does not cause motility disturbance if preseptal
E   more frequently causes complications in children than in adults

Conjunctiva and cornea

127. Extreme photophobia is characteristic of:

A   homocystinuria
B   cystinosis
C   aniridia
D   mycotic keratitis
E   *Acanthamoeba* keratitis

128. Down's syndrome is

A   associated with keratoconus
B   associated with blepharitis
C   associated with myopia
D   associated with a higher chance of recurrence in a sibling if the
     mother is a balanced translocation carrier than if due to
     non-dysjunction
E   due to trisomy 18

129. Terrien's disease typically

A   is unilateral
B   leads to loss of epithelium
C   causes visual impairment due to astigmatism
D   is painless
E   affects females

130. The finding of eosinophils on conjunctival cytology is a feature of:

A   molluscum contagiosum
B   vernal disease
C   hayfever conjunctivitis
D   mucous membrane pemphigoid
E   adult chlamydial infection

131. The following cause a follicular conjunctival reaction:

A   molluscum contagiosum
B   *Moraxella lacunata*
C   trachoma
D   adenovirus
E   vernal keratoconjunctivitis

132. **Subconjunctival haemorrhage is a typical feature of:**

A   blood dyscrasias
B   picornavirus conjunctivitis
C   adenovirus conjunctivitis
D   *Haemophilus* conjunctivitis
E   subarachnoid haemorrhage

133. **Differential diagnosis for a membranous or pseudomembranous conjunctivitis includes:**

A   Stevens-Johnson syndrome
B   primary Herpes simplex infection
C   gonococcus infection
D   *Moraxella* infection
E   ligneous conjunctivitis

134. **Giant conjunctival papillae occur in:**

A   ocular prosthesis wear
B   palpebral vernal conjunctivitis
C   *Acanthamoeba* infection
D   drug preservative toxicity
E   adenovirus conjunctivitis

135. **Differential diagnosis for a corneal pannus includes:**

A   Thygeson's (superficial punctate) keratitis
B   rosacea keratitis
C   fungal keratitis
D   Herpes zoster
E   trachoma

136. **Filamentary keratitis is a recognised feature of:**

A   Herpes simplex keratitis
B   Herpes zoster keratitis
C   superior limbic keratoconjunctivitis
D   amiodarone keratopathy
E   keratoconjunctivitis sicca

137. **Clinical features of ophthalmic herpes zoster include:**

A   mucous plaque keratitis
B   scleritis
C   ring-shaped corneal infiltrate
D   entropion
E   mucopurulent conjunctivitis

138. **Band keratopathy is**

A caused by stromal deposition of calcium salts
B characteristically separated from the limbus by a clear space
C seen in an otherwise normal eye in an elderly patient
D seen in renal failure
E treated by lamellar keratoplasty

139. **Recurrent corneal erosions frequently occur in**

A Salzmann's nodular degeneration
B granular dystrophy
C lattice dystrophy
D keratoglobus
E Reis–Bücklers' dystrophy

140. **The following statements about keratoconus are true:**

A spherical and astigmatic refractive error results
B corneal perforation is a feature
C prominent corneal nerves are seen early in disease
D prognosis following keratoplasty is excellent
E asthma is associated

141. **Climatic keratopathy**

A is more common in females
B is associated with cumulative exposure to infrared light
C is associated with vascularisation
D is associated with anterior lens capsule changes
E affects the anterior stroma

142. **Penetrating keratoplasty has, in general, a good prognosis in the following disorders:**

A keratoconus
B Fuchs' endothelial dystrophy
C chemical burns
D Herpes simplex keratitis
E Stevens–Johnson syndrome

143. **Acute haemorrhagic conjunctivitis**

A is caused by picornaviruses
B is unilateral at onset
C may be treated with specific antimicrobial agents
D causes keratitis very rarely
E is asymptomatic in most patients

144. **Adult inclusion conjunctivitis**

A   is caused by adenovirus
B   causes nummular subepithelial lesions
C   causes pannus
D   is usually unilateral
E   responds well to topical corticosteroids

145. **The following statements about trachoma are true:**

A   in developing countries, it is seen more commonly in urban than rural populations
B   in the acute phase, conjunctival papillae are seen
C   in the acute phase, conjunctival follicles are seen
D   vaccination is used in prevention
E   Giemsa stain is useful in diagnosis

146. **Vernal keratoconjunctivitis:**

A   is much more common in males
B   is often asymmetrical
C   esotropia is a recognised sequel
D   is caused by contact lens wear in some patients
E   is seen in non-atopic subjects

147. **The following statements about cicatrising conjunctivitis are true:**

A   Stevens–Johnson syndrome is the commonest cause
B   practolol is the drug most commonly implicated
C   it is associated with pseudomembrane formation
D   it causes lagophthalmos
E   surgical treatment of symblepharon with mucous membrane grafts is usually successful

148. **Pterygium**

A   occurs in Terrien's marginal degeneration
B   may extend deep to Bowman's layer
C   causes diminished visual acuity in some cases
D   causes restricted ocular motility in some cases
E   may be a manifestation of topical drug toxicity

149. **The following statements about conjunctival flap surgery are true:**

A   it is useful in neurotrophic corneal ulceration
B   it is useful in corneal perforation
C   ptosis is a complication
D   infection of the flap is the most common complication
E   therapeutic bandage contact lenses are an alternative therapy

150. **Epibulbar dermoids**

A   are most often located at the inferotemporal limbus
B   have malignant potential
C   may be associated with colobomas
D   may be hereditary
E   are covered by conjunctival epithelium

151. **Features of acne rosacea include:**

A   scarring pustules
B   recurrent corneal epithelial erosions
C   corneal perforation
D   response to systemic tetracycline
E   response to systemic erythromycin

152. **The following conjunctival lesions commonly undergo malignant transformation:**

A   conjunctival epithelial melanosis
B   congenital melanosis oculi
C   primary acquired melanosis
D   secondary acquired melanosis
E   papilloma

153. **Surgical procedures used in the management of malignant melanoma of the conjunctiva include:**

A   biopsy
B   enucleation
C   exenteration
D   cryotherapy
E   diathermy

Glaucoma

154. **The following are features of pseudoexfoliation syndrome:**

A   zonule weakness
B   pale of absent trabecular meshwork pigmentation
C   iridocapsular adhesions
D   incomplete response to mydriatics
E   open-angle glaucoma in most patients

155. **Pigmentation of the trabecular meshwork**

A   decreases with age
B   is more marked in patients with darkly pigmented irides
C   is more marked in the inferior angle
D   is increased in Fuchs' heterochromic cyclitis
E   is decreased in pigment dispersion syndrome

156. **The following ophthalmoscopic signs suggest glaucoma:**

A   symmetrical cups
B   disc haemorrhage
C   absent disc venous pulsation
D   narrowing of the neuroretinal rim
E   vertical elongation of the cup

157. **The following statements about the anterior chamber angle are true:**

A   Schwalbe's line is situated posterior to the trabecular meshwork
B   the scleral spur is situated posterior to the trabecular meshwork
C   pigmentation of the trabecular meshwork is rare in childhood
D   Schlemm's canal is usually visible on gonioscopy
E   the ciliary body is usually visible on gonioscopy

158. **The following are recognised to occur after trabeculectomy:**

A   corneal pigmentation
B   ciliary block glaucoma
C   continuing loss of visual field if intraocular pressure control is satisfactory
D   retinal detachment
E   choroidal detachment

159. Primary angle-closure glaucoma

A   is more prevalent than open-angle glaucoma in Europe
B   is more prevalent than open-angle glaucoma in South-East Asia
C   is treated in some cases by trabeculectomy
D   causes disc cupping
E   causes ischaemic optic neuropathy

160. Increased intraocular pressure is a recognised feature of:

A   benign intracranial hypertension
B   Leber's hereditary optic neuropathy
C   interstitial keratitis
D   dysthyroid eye disease
E   dural cavernous fistula

161. In nanophthalmos, the

A   corneal diameter is typically normal
B   axial length of the eye is shortened
C   eye is susceptible to open-angle glaucoma
D   sclera is abnormally thin
E   incidence of retinal detachment is high

162. The following disorders are associated with neovascular glaucoma:

A   caroticocavernous fistula
B   branch retinal vein occlusion
C   ischaemic optic neuropathy
D   background diabetic retinopathy
E   Coats' disease

163. You are asked to manage a patient with rubeosis iridis. The following statements are true:

A   if iris neovascularisation is evident, cyclocryotherapy is the treatment of choice
B   panretinal photocoagulation should be attempted, even if there is synechial angle closure
C   trabeculectomy will lower intraocular pressure if neovascularisation can be induced to regress
D   if the eye is painful and blind, evisceration is the treatment of choice
E   aqueous flare is consistent with the diagnosis of neovascular glaucoma

164. **The following are associated with angle-closure glaucoma:**

A glaucomatocyclitic crisis (Posner–Schlossman syndrome)
B persistent hyperplastic primary vitreous
C epithelial ingrowth complicating cataract surgery
D traumatic angle recession
E phacomorphic glaucoma

165. **Features of the iridocorneal endothelial (ICE) syndromes include:**

A posterior embryotoxon
B iris strands to Schwalbe's line
C iris stromal atrophy
D open-angle glaucoma
E onset in childhood

166. **Primary congenital glaucoma (buphthalmos)**

A is unilateral in most cases
B is associated with abnormalities of Descemet's membrane
C does not cause disc cupping
D responds poorly to medical treatment
E is associated with normal findings on gonioscopy

167. **Aniridia is associated with:**

A foveal hypoplasia
B corneal pannus
C renal malignancy in hereditary rather than sporadic cases
D onset of Wilms' tumour before 2 years of age
E difficulty of intraocular pressure control in glaucoma cases

168. **Rieger's syndrome is characterised by:**

A recessive inheritance
B posterior embryotoxon
C corneal opacity
D lens opacity
E iris stromal hypoplasia

Lens

169. In the presence of a mature cataract but an otherwise normal eye

A   light perception should be brisk and unequivocal
B   light perception without projection may be found
C   an afferent pupil defect may be found
D   visual field testing is uninformative if visual acuity is less than counting fingers
E   the photostress test is useful in evaluation

170. Cataract occurs in:

A   long-term chloroquine treatment
B   long-term busulphan treatment
C   hyperparathyroidism
D   Duchenne muscular dystrophy
E   atopic dermatitis

171. In extracapsular cataract extraction, potential complications of irrigation and aspiration include:

A   zonular dehiscence
B   detachment of Descemet's membrane
C   endophthalmitis
D   hyphaema
E   lens cortex loss into the vitreous humour

172. Endocapsular cataract extraction

A   is contraindicated in lens dislocation
B   requires a smaller surgical section than extracapsular extraction
C   cannot be combined with phacoemulsification
D   involves anterior lens capsule removal prior to IOL insertion
E   affords more protection to the posterior capsule than extracapsular extraction

173. **Advantages of extracapsular extraction over intracapsular extraction include:**

A less corneal endothelial cell loss
B less vitreous loss
C better corrected Snellen visual acuity in uncomplicated cases
D lower incidence of cystoid macular oedema
E faster surgical procedure

174. **The following statements about congenital cataract are true:**

A about half the cases are genetically determined
B genetically determined cataract is usually associated with other ocular abnormalities
C isolated hereditary cataract is most commonly autosomal dominant
D underlying systemic disease will be found in the majority
E as a general rule, cataract is removed from the eye with better vision first

175. **Posterior subcapsular cataract**

A is typical of drug-induced lens opacity
B is the type of cataract typically found in Wilson's disease
C causes glare symptoms less often than cortical cataract
D affects distance before near vision
E is the most common type of lens opacity affecting patients less than 60 years old

176. **Cataract may be associated with:**

A ecothiopate
B prednisolone
C chlorpropamide
D cornea verticillata
E subnormal scotopic ERG amplitude

177. **Factors leading to raised intraocular pressure following cataract extraction include:**

A vitreous touch syndrome
B use of α-chymotrypsin
C choroidal detachment
D epithelial ingrowth
E residual lens cortex

178. **Endophthalmitis following cataract extraction is**

A   most commonly caused by *Staphylococcus aureus*
B   caused by anaerobic bacteria
C   caused by fungi
D   invariably caused by microbial infection
E   treated with parenteral antibiotics

179. **Rupture of the posterior capsule during extracapsular cataract extraction**

A   is the commonest cause of vitreous loss in that operation
B   if accompanied by displacement of vitreous into the anterior chamber should be managed by anterior vitrectomy
C   is a contraindication to posterior chamber lens implantation
D   indicates that no further lens cortex should be aspirated
E   is performed in some cases as a primary procedure

180. **Non-traumatic lens subluxation occurs in:**

A   hyperornithinaemia
B   buphthalmos
C   high myopia
D   hyperlysinaemia
E   dystrophia myotonica

181. **Difficulties encountered at extracapsular cataract extraction that are characteristic of pseudoexfoliation syndrome include:**

A   poor pupil dilation
B   corneal oedema
C   hyphaema
D   zonule dehiscence
E   unstable intraocular pressure

182. **Nd–YAG laser posterior capsulotomy**

A   causes intraocular pressure increase, maximal on the following day
B   –induced lens implant damage is usually symptomatic
C   may lead to epithelial downgrowth
D   may lead to anterior hyaloid face rupture
E   if indicated, is ideally performed within 6 months of surgery

183. **The following are recognised causes of cataract:**

A   infrared radiation
B   ultraviolet radiation
C   microwaves
D   uncomplicated strabismus surgery
E   uncomplicated trabeculectomy

Uveal tract

184. **Heterochromia iridis may be seen in a patient with:**

A   ptosis
B   incontinentia pigmenti
C   Sturge–Weber syndrome
D   acute leukaemia
E   intraocular foreign body

185. **In juvenile chronic arthritis:**

A   uveitis is more common in the polyarticular group
B   uveitis is accompanied by discomfort and redness
C   rheumatoid factor is positive
D   macular oedema is a cause of visual loss
E   Salzmann's nodular degeneration is a feature

186. **In Reiter's syndrome:**

A   almost all patients are male
B   HLA-B27 is positive in 50%
C   uveitis is more common than conjunctivitis
D   the conjunctival reaction is usually papillary
E   patients usually develop chronic arthritis

187. **In ankylosing spondylitis:**

A   most patients develop uveitis
B   HLA–B27 is positive in 50%
C   rheumatoid factor usually positive
D   conjunctivitis is a common feature
E   the joints of the lumbar spine are the first to be affected

188. **Vogt–Koyanagi–Harada disease typically**

A involves both eyes
B involves the choriocapillaris
C is associated with skin abnormalities
D gives rise to Touton giant cells in involved tissue
E causes meningeal inflammation

189. **A patient presents with anterior uveitis, arthritis and erythema nodosum. The following are possible diagnoses:**

A Behçet's disease
B sarcoidosis
C Crohn's disease
D Reiter's disease
E leprosy

190. **The following may be seen in a patient with productive cough and a positive Mantoux test:**

A granulomatous anterior uveitis
B non-granulomatous anterior uveitis
C scattered pale lesions on fundoscopy
D optic neuropathy
E phlyctenulosis

191. **Features of Fuchs' heterochromic cyclitis include:**

A diffusely scattered pigmented keratic precipitates
B posterior synechiae
C iris vascular occlusion
D glaucoma
E unilateral disease in all cases

192. **Ocular manifestations of acquired immune deficiency syndrome include:**

A Herpes zoster ophthalmicus
B retinal haemorrhages
C nerve fibre layer infarcts
D hyphaema
E unilateral optic disc swelling

193. **In presumed ocular histoplasmosis syndrome (POHS):**

A   anterior uveitis occurs
B   there are multifocal atrophic choroidal lesions
C   breaks in Bruch's membrane occur
D   antifungal agents are effective in therapy
E   many patients are intravenous drug abusers

194. *Toxoplasma gondii*

A   is an extracellular parasite
B   oöcytes are spread by dogs
C   causes intraocular calcification
D   infection is recent if the dye test is positive
E   retinochoroiditis is treated by oral clindamycin

195. **The following cause multifocal choroiditis:**

A   *Nocardia asteroides*
B   presumed ocular histoplasmosis syndrome
C   tuberculosis
D   ankylosing spondylitis
E   measles

196. **In onchocerciasis:**

A   inflammation is caused by live worms
B   microfilariae are visible on slit lamp examination
C   ivermectin is the treatment of choice
D   extraocular disease manifestations are uncommon
E   optic atrophy occurs

197. **In sarcoidosis:**

A   anterior uveitis is the commonest ocular abnormality
B   retinal arteritis is typical
C   caseating granuloma is the characteristic pathological sign
D   optic disc swelling implies CNS involvement
E   Kveim antigen skin testing frequently causes exacerbation
    of ocular inflammation

198. **Malignant melanoma of the iris**

A   causes cataract
B   is composed of spindle cell types in almost all cases
C   is treated by enucleation in some cases
D   is more common than ciliary body melanoma
E   has an excellent prognosis

199. **The following statements about postoperative endophthalmitis are true:**

A   *Pseudomonas aeruginosa* is the commonest causative organism
B   in fungal endophthalmitis, the onset of signs is delayed characteristically until at least three weeks after surgery
C   anaerobic bacteria do not cause intraocular infection
D   lid oedema is typical
E   pyrexia does not occur

200. **The following statements about choroidal melanoma are true:**

A   it is more radiosensitive than retinoblastoma
B   it may be distinguished from choroidal haemangioma by the presence of secondary serous retinal detachment
C   the lung is the second most common initial site of metastases
D   primary treatment in some cases may be chemotherapy
E   primary treatment in some cases may be laser photocoagulation

201. **The following statements about intraocular tumours are true:**

A   medulloepithelioma arises from the retinal pigment epithelium
B   choroidal osteoma typically arises from the juxtapapillary choroid
C   uveal malignant melanoma is more common in black than white races
D   melanocytoma does not produce visual field defects
E   melanocytoma has minimal malignant potential

202. **Choroidal haemangioma**

A   of diffuse type may be associated with meningeal angioma
B   of nodular type may be associated with neurofibromatosis
C   is usually situated in the periphery
D   causes choroidal folds
E   treatment by laser photocoagulation is dangerous

203. Choroidal metastatic tumours

A in some cases cause extensive serous detachment of neurosensory retina
B arise most commonly from the gastrointestinal tract in male patients
C seldom become significantly elevated
D are less common than orbital metastases
E are best treated by radiotherapy if central vision is threatened

Vitreous and retina

204. Retinal haemorrhages occur

A in normal neonates
B at high altitude
C in diabetic maculopathy without proliferative retinopathy
D with raised intracranial pressure
E in sickle-cell haemoglobin C disease

205. Posterior scleritis is

A usually associated with systemic disease
B associated with choroidal detachment
C associated with retinal detachment
D diagnosed by ultrasonography
E not treated in the same way as anterior scleritis

206. In retinitis pigmentosa:

A narrowing of retinal vessels is typical
B autosomal dominant inheritance is most common
C with X-linked inheritance, the disease follows a relatively benign course
D lamellar macular holes occur
E epiretinal membranes occur

207. **The following statements about electrodiagnostic tests in retinitis pigmentosa are true:**

A   the photopic ERG is relatively unaffected
B   the ERG may be extinguished in the absence of field loss
C   the EOG is normal
D   dark adaptation shows elevation of cone and rod thresholds
E   the VER is unaffected

208. **The following statements are true:**

A   Refsum's disease causes deafness and pigmentary retinopathy
B   abetalipoproteinaemia is treated with vitamin E
C   in Leber's congenital amaurosis, the diagnosis is made on the basis of an abnormal VER
D   in Leber's congenital amaurosis, photophobia is typical
E   gyrate atrophy is due to increased levels of phytanic acid

209. **In choroideraemia:**

A   inheritance is autosomal recessive
B   central vision is affected earlier than peripheral vision
C   retinal blood vessels are typically attenuated
D   choroidal pigment migrates forward into the anterior layers of the retina
E   the ERG is normal

210. **In Best's macular dystrophy:**

A   visual acuity correlates with electrodiagnostic changes
B   visual acuity is normal until the vitelliruptive ('scrambled egg') stage
C   inheritance is X-linked
D   ERG is the electrodiagnostic test of choice
E   electrodiagnostic abnormalities are found in carriers with normal fundi

211. **The following are typical findings in ocular albinism:**

A   normal number of melanocytes
B   pendular nystagmus
C   orthophoria
D   emmetropia
E   melanosomes on skin biopsy

212. **The Snellen visual acuity given below would be expected in the condition named:**

A   6/60 (20/200) with a true macular hole
B   6/24 (20/80) in tyrosinase-positive oculocutaneous albinism
C   6/60 (20/200) in central serous choroidopathy
D   < 6/60 (20/200) in arteritic ischaemic optic neuropathy
E   6/6 (20/20) in melanocytoma of the optic disc

213. **The following retinal lesions should be treated with prophylactic cryopexy:**

A   holes at the vitreous base
B   large U-shaped break, with vitreous attached to the flap but no subretinal fluid, in the eye of a patient with symptoms of acute posterior vitreous detachment
C   holes in the inner layer of acquired retinoschisis
D   snail track degeneration
E   pavingstone degeneration

214. **Causes of exudative retinal detachment include:**

A   renal failure
B   proliferative retinopathy
C   Harada's disease
D   uveal melanoma
E   penetrating ocular trauma

215. **The following statements about persistent hyperplastic primary vitreous (PHPV) are correct:**

A   posterior PHPV is the most common type
B   PHPV typically occurs in an otherwise normal eye
C   PHPV is usually bilateral
D   ciliary processes are abnormal
E   prognosis for vision is good in anterior PHPV

216. **Complications of argon laser photocoagulation include:**

A   defective colour vision
B   choroidal haemorrhage
C   retinal haemorrhage
D   retinal nerve fibre bundle defects
E   raised intraocular pressure

217. **Argon laser photocoagulation may be beneficial in the following conditions:**

A rubeosis iridis
B ischaemic diabetic maculopathy
C exudative diabetic maculopathy
D oedematous diabetic maculopathy
E central serous choroidopathy

218. **Severe ocular complications occur in**

A sickle-cell haemoglobin C (SC) disease
B sickle-cell anaemia (SS)
C sickle-cell thalassaemia (SThal)
D abetalipoproteinaemia
E retinopathy of prematurity, stage 2

219. **Features of sickle-cell eye disease include:**

A traction retinal detachment
B elevated new vessels
C anterior segment ischaemia
D cystoid macular oedema
E iris atrophy

220. **Features of cicatricial retinopathy of prematurity include:**

A optic atrophy
B ectopia lentis
C strabismus
D ectopia of macula
E optic nerve hypoplasia

221. **Drüsen**

A are located between the retinal pigment epithelium and the neurosensory retina
B undergo secondary calcification
C cause peripapillary haemorrhage
D may cause visual loss without the formation of a subretinal neovascular membrane or RPE changes
E are associated with ERG changes

222. **Subretinal neovascular membranes may be managed by laser photocoagulation if**

A visual acuity is 6/60 (20/200)
B 300 μm from foveola on fluorescein angiogram
C associated with RPE detachment
D central vision in the other eye has been lost due to macular degeneration
E krypton laser is not available

223. **In central serous choroidopathy:**

A elevation of neurosensory retina is accompanied by underlying RPE detachment
B duration of elevation of neurosensory retina correlates with final vision
C the recurrence rate is 40%
D females are typically affected
E optic nerve hypoplasia may be associated

224. **Purtscher's retinopathy**

A follows long bone fractures
B follows chest compression injuries
C is characterised by florid haemorrhages in the nerve fibre layer
D is characterised by scattered cotton wool patches
E has a bad prognosis

225. **The following are recognised associations of cystoid macular oedema:**

A epiretinal membrane
B tamoxifen
C argon laser photocoagulation
D family history
E choroideraemia

226. **In X-linked retinoschisis:**

A visual acuity becomes progressively impaired
B the ERG is normal
C the EOG is normal
D vitreous haemorrhage occurs
E the optic disc is typically abnormal

227. **Angioid streaks are**

A   due to breaks in the RPE
B   hyperfluorescent on fluorescein angiography
C   associated with rupture of choroid
D   associated with multiple myeloma
E   associated with Ehlers–Danlos syndrome

228. **The following cause maculopathy:**

A   gold
B   quinine
C   chlorpromazine
D   thioridazine
E   subacute sclerosing panencephalitis

229. **Regarding a child with bilateral retinoblastoma, the following statements are correct:**

A   bilaterality implies that the tumour is inherited
B   if a sibling is also affected, the risk of subsequent children being affected is 25%
C   if the child survives, there is a 6% chance that his children will develop the tumour
D   age at diagnosis is similar in bilateral and unilateral cases
E   the liver is the most likely site of metastases

230. **Retinal astrocytoma**

A   is associated with epilepsy
B   is treated with photocoagulation
C   may be a feature of Sturge–Weber syndrome
D   is associated with CNS tumour
E   is associated with café-au-lait spots

231. **Silicone oil in conjunction with pars plana vitrectomy**

A   is used in the treatment of uncomplicated rhegmatogenous retinal detachment
B   is used in the treatment of proliferative vitreoretinopathy
C   contraindicates further laser photocoagulation
D   is frequently complicated by cataract in phakic patients
E   is frequently complicated by band keratopathy

232. **The following are signs of preproliferative diabetic retinopathy:**

A   intraretinal microvascular abnormalities
B   fibrovascular membranes
C   cotton wool patches
D   retinal detachment
E   non-arteritic ischaemic optic neuropathy

233. **Typical (senile adult) retinoschisis**

A   is inferotemporal in 70%
B   is usually bilateral
C   is X-linked
D   is associated with maculopathy
E   tends not to progress posteriorly

Motility

234. **Recession of**

A   a vertical muscle has a greater effect than recession of a horizontal muscle
B   lateral rectus has a greater effect than recession of medial rectus
C   both medial recti is indicated in divergence insufficiency esodeviation
D   both lateral recti is indicated in divergence excess exodeviation
E   conjunctiva increases the effect of muscle recession

235. **In strabismus surgery:**

A   non-absorbable material must be used for suture of muscle to sclera
B   in children, Tenon's capsule is easily dissected as a separate layer from the conjunctiva
C   limitation of ocular movements results from resection of more than 5.5 mm of lateral rectus
D   the inferior oblique is approached and exposed through the inferonasal fornix
E   the superior oblique is approached at the lateral margin of the superior rectus

236. **Adjustable suture surgery is**

A   more suitable for resection than recession of muscles
B   more suitable for vertical than horizontal recti
C   suitable in children
D   unsuitable in dysthyroid ophthalmopathy
E   unsuitable in re-operations

237. **Worth's four-dot test**

A   is performed for near and distance
B   may be used to diagnose microtropia (monofixation syndrome)
C   may be used to diagnose anomalous retinal correspondence (ARC)
D   indicates binocular vision if the patient sees five lights
E   indicates diplopia if the patient sees alternating red and green lights

238. **Which of the following have secondary abducting action?**

A   superior rectus
B   superior oblique
C   inferior rectus
D   inferior oblique
E   none of the above

239. **The following statements about testing of ocular motility are correct:**

A   a prism is held base out in measurement of a divergent squint
B   the Maddox wing test measures heterophoria
C   the Maddox rod test is used to measure vertical deviations
D   the 4 dioptre prism test is used to identify simultaneous perception
E   if in the Bielschowsky head tilting test an upshoot is seen, this implies a superior rectus palsy in that eye

240. **In infantile (congenital) esotropia:**

A   the infant is excessively hypermetropic
B   latent nystagmus is a feature
C   dissociated vertical deviation is a feature
D   the angle of deviation is similar for near and distance
E   cross-fixating infants should receive occlusion treatment

241. **In microtropia (monofixation syndrome):**

A binocular single vision is absent
B esodeviation is usual
C amblyopia is not a feature
D a central scotoma is always present
E eccentric fixation is a feature

242. **The following may be used to test stereopsis:**

A TNO test
B Worth's four-dot test
C synoptophore
D bar reading
E Bagolini striated glasses

243. **In convergence excess esotropia:**

A an AC/A ratio of 3:1 is typical
B amblyopia is common
C bifocal spectacles are an effective form of treatment
D ecothiopate (Phospholine Iodide) is used
E surgery is confined to the medial recti

244. **Faden (posterior fixation) sutures**

A augment resection of muscle
B must be nonabsorbable and permanent
C are used only on rectus muscles
D are indicated in dissociated vertical deviation (DVD)
E are of no value in paralytic strabismus

245. **Inferior oblique overaction**

A gives rise to an A pattern
B causes concomitant strabismus
C if treated by a weakening procedure may reduce the horizontal esodeviation
D is more commonly bilateral than unilateral
E is treated by myectomy

246. **Intermittent exotropia**

A   is commoner than constant primary exotropia
B   of the divergence excess type is controlled for near fixation
C   of the divergence excess type is characterised by normal convergence
D   of the divergence excess type is treated in some cases by concave lenses
E   is associated with mental retardation

247. **Duane's retraction syndrome**

A   is usually bilateral
B   rarely causes diplopia
C   patients do not have binocular single vision
D   causes esotropia in most patients with the disorder
E   requires surgical treatment in most cases

248. **In Brown's syndrome:**

A   the Hess chart shows no abnormality in the upper field
B   eye movements simulate superior oblique palsy
C   treatment is unnecessary in most patients
D   the abnormality tends to worsen with age
E   a deviation in primary position is usual

Neuro-ophthalmology

249. **Uniocular diplopia occurs in:**

A   lens opacity
B   peripheral iridectomy
C   iridodialysis
D   optic nerve lesion
E   chiasm compression

250. **The following statements about pupil reactions are correct:**

A   physiological anisocoria is distinguishable in 20%
B   the difference in pupil size in physiological anisocoria is unequal in light and dark
C   cocaine drops are used in the differential diagnosis of a dilated pupil
D   pilocarpine drops are used in the differential diagnosis of a dilated pupil
E   hydroxyamphetamine drops are used in the differential diagnosis of a dilated pupil

251. **In complete afferent pupil defect:**

A   no consensual reflex is seen in the affected eye
B   no consensual reflex is seen in the fellow eye
C   no direct reflex is seen in the affected eye
D   an optic nerve lesion is a possible diagnosis
E   an occipital cortex lesion is a possible diagnosis

252. **The following may cause Horner's syndrome:**

A   subclavian artery aneurysm
B   caroticocavernous fistula
C   thyroid disease
D   cervical rib
E   demyelination

253. **Features of Argyll Robertson pupil include:**

A   no light reflex
B   no near reflex
C   dilation with cocaine
D   iris atrophy
E   usually unilateral

254. **Optic nerve pallor is seen in:**

A   a lesion of the optic tract
B   a lesion of the optic radiation
C   retinitis pigmentosa
D   mucopolysaccharidosis
E   neurofibromatosis

255. **Spasmus nutans**

A   is a cause of abnormal head posture
B   typically starts at about 3 years of age
C   may occur in adults
D   causes nystagmus
E   is usually binocular

256. **Uniocular nystagmus is seen in:**

A   internuclear ophthalmoplegia
B   infantile esotropia syndrome
C   drug toxicity
D   cerebellar disease
E   spasmus nutans

257. The following cause upbeat vertical nystagmus:

A Arnold-Chiari malformation
B internuclear ophthalmoplegia
C anticonvulsant drugs
D cerebellar disease
E lesion in the dorsal midbrain

258. Concerning the third cranial nerve:

A its nucleus is situated dorsal to the aqueduct
B innervation of the superior rectus is contralateral
C a nuclear lesion causes bilateral ptosis
D palsy may cause proptosis
E it may be involved in migraine

259. Sixth cranial nerve palsy may be associated with

A dorsal midbrain lesion
B raised intraocular pressure
C ear infection
D nasopharyngeal carcinoma
E rubella

260. Tolosa-Hunt syndrome

A causes proptosis
B causes pain
C does not respond to corticosteroid
D is diagnosed by angiography
E causes abnormal eye movements

261. Internuclear ophthalmoplegia

A usually causes diplopia
B affects convergence
C is usually caused by demyelination
D causes nystagmus
E is usually accompanied by sixth cranial nerve palsy

262. Horizontal gaze palsy

A is caused by a midbrain lesion
B is caused by a pontine lesion
C is usually bilateral
D usually affects convergence
E in an elderly patient is usually caused by a tumour

263. **In benign intracranial hypertension:**

A   no visual symptoms occur
B   optic disc swelling occurs
C   diplopia occurs
D   CT brain scan is normal
E   spontaneous recovery occurs

264. **Seventh cranial nerve palsy**

A   of lower motor neuron type causes a dry exposed eye
B   of upper motor neuron type causes a dry exposed eye
C   may be associated with hemiplegia
D   may be associated with herpes zoster
E   may be associated with acoustic neuroma

265. **A lesion in the cerebellopontine angle causes**

A   a dry eye
B   corneal anaesthesia
C   lagophthalmos
D   deafness
E   third cranial nerve palsy

266. **Lid retraction occurs in:**

A   Horner's syndrome
B   sympathetic overaction
C   dysthyroid eye disease
D   dorsal midbrain syndrome
E   demyelination

267. **The following are features of dorsal midbrain syndrome:**

A   nystagmus
B   Adie pupil
C   disturbance of vertical gaze
D   third cranial nerve palsy
E   optic nerve pallor

268. **The following are seen in early papilloedema:**

A   retinal exudates
B   enlarged blind spot in visual field
C   loss of venous pulsation
D   choroidal folds
E   optic disc pallor

269. **Optic neuritis**

A   may be associated with viral infection
B   may be associated with demyelination
C   causes an altitudinal field defect
D   is often asymptomatic
E   is best diagnosed by ERG

270. **Optic disc drüsen**

A   may be diagnosed by CT scan
B   cause optic disc cupping
C   cause visual field defects
D   may cause haemorrhage
E   may mimic papilloedema

271. **Features of oculomotor apraxia include:**

A   abnormal pursuit eye movements
B   abnormal saccadic eye movements
C   abnormal vestibulo-ocular reflex
D   blindness
E   head thrusts

272. **A patient presents with acute third cranial nerve palsy due to a lesion within the ventral midbrain. The following signs would be expected:**

A   convergence–retraction nystagmus
B   ipsilateral hemiparesis
C   contralateral choreoathetosis
D   complete ptosis
E   normal pupil reactions if the lesion is in the nucleus

273. **In Steele–Richardson disease**

A   doll's head reflexes are lost first
B   pursuit movements are lost before saccadic movements
C   horizontal gaze is affected
D   dementia occurs
E   young adults are affected

274. **Fourth cranial nerve**

A   nucleus is situated posterior to the aqueduct of Silvius
B   decussates
C   palsy seldom indicates serious neurological disease
D   palsy is most commonly due to vascular disease
E   palsy is the cause of Brown's syndrome

275. **The following forms of nystagmus are pathological:**

A   optokinetic nystagmus
B   end-point
C   periodic alternating nystagmus
D   gaze-evoked
E   upbeat in upgaze

276. **Features of Wernicke–Korsakoff syndrome include:**

A   vertical gaze paresis
B   fourth cranial nerve palsy
C   retinal haemorrhages
D   nystagmus
E   response to pyridoxine (vitamin B_6)

277. **Complete loss of right optic tract function is associated with**

A   homonymous hemianopia
B   left afferent pupil defect
C   normal colour vision in the left eye
D   normal visual acuity in the left eye
E   optic atrophy

278. **Miosis is a feature of**

A   leprosy
B   Adie pupil
C   pontine haemorrhage
D   midbrain haemorrhage
E   opiate overdose

Neurology and systemic diseases

279. Features of posterior inferior cerebellar artery thrombosis include:

A   ipsilateral corneal anaesthesia
B   horizontal jerk nystagmus to ipsilateral side
C   contralateral sensory loss of limbs to pain
D   sudden onset of vertigo
E   ipsilateral Horner's syndrome

280. Posterior cerebral artery thrombosis causes

A   hemianopia
B   nominal aphasia
C   contralateral hemihypaesthesia
D   apractagnosia
E   sensory ataxia

281. Cerebellar disease causes

A   dysphasia
B   dysarthria
C   nystagmus
D   sensory ataxia
E   limb weakness

282. In Behçet's disease

A   retinal arteries are more often affected than veins
B   retinal neovascularisation is a feature
C   mild anterior uveitis is typical
D   laboratory tests are unhelpful in diagnosis
E   oral cyclosporin A is the treatment of choice

283. Features of Sturge–Weber syndrome include

A   cataract
B   glaucoma
C   convulsions
D   hemianopia
E   mental retardation

284. **Wilson's disease**

A is associated with cataract
B is associated with retinopathy
C is diagnosed by the finding of a high total serum copper level
D inheritance is autosomal dominant
E Kayser–Fleischer ring disappears on treatment with penicillamine

285. **Congenital toxoplasmosis causes**

A hydrocephalus
B microphthalmos
C vitritis
D cervical lymphadenopathy
E seizure disorder

286. **Chronic sarcoidosis, unlike the acute presentation, is characterised by**

A bihilar lymphadenopathy on chest X-ray
B erythema nodosum
C increased serum angiotensin converting enzyme
D hypercalcaemia
E impaired humoral immunity

287. **In giant cell arteritis:**

A those vessels without an internal elastic lamina are preferentially affected
B pathological changes are limited to the arteries of the head and neck
C ischaemic optic neuropathy is more common than central retinal artery occlusion
D elevated haemoglobin is often found in the acute phase of the disease
E pain on mastication is a highly suggestive symptom

288. **The following statements about onchocerciasis are correct:**

A most blindness due to this disease occurs in central Africa
B ocular inflammation is caused by the dead microfilariae
C it causes intense pruritus
D it causes optic atrophy
E ivermectin is the microfilaricide of choice in therapy

289. **Glucose intolerance is associated with:**

A   retinitis pigmentosa
B   systemic glucocorticoid therapy
C   sixth cranial nerve palsy in an elderly patient
D   pituitary adenoma secreting growth hormone
E   Friedreich's ataxia

290. **Ocular findings typical of leprosy include:**

A   raised intraocular pressure
B   cataract
C   anterior uveitis
D   blepharospasm
E   reduced corneal sensation

291. **The following occur in congenital rubella infection:**

A   maculopathy
B   bilateral cataract
C   glaucoma
D   thrombocytopenia
E   cyanotic congenital heart disease

292. **Dystrophia myotonica**

A   affects only males
B   causes testicular atrophy
C   causes cardiac abnormalities
D   causes ptosis more commonly than lens opacity
E   causes pigmentary retinopathy

293. **Features of atopic dermatitis include:**

A   retinal detachment
B   anterior subcapsular cataract
C   corneal opacity
D   abnormally high IgA levels
E   susceptibility to herpes simplex infections

294. **Features of classic galactosaemia include:**

A   hypoglycaemia
B   normal IQ
C   dislocated lens
D   reversible lens opacity
E   diagnosis by examination of urine for non-glucose reducing sugar

295. **The following cause deafness and ocular disorder:**

A   DIDMOAD syndrome
B   congenital syphilis
C   Alport's syndrome
D   Vogt–Koyanagi–Harada syndrome
E   Usher's syndrome

296. **In Laurence–Moon–Biedl syndrome:**

A   inheritance is autosomal dominant
B   truncal obesity occurs
C   IQ is within the normal range
D   marked ERG changes may be evident in the absence of clinical retinal disease
E   severe renal disease is typical

297. **In multiple sclerosis:**

A   the oligodendrocyte nucleus is affected
B   the oligodendrocyte myelin component is affected
C   the Schwann cell myelin is affected
D   gliosis occurs
E   optic neuritis occurs in most patients

298. **The following are typical of occipital cortex lesions:**

A   visual inattention
B   incongruous field defects
C   macular sparing
D   relative afferent pupil defect
E   abnormal saccadic eye movements

299. **Craniopharyngioma**

A usually occurs in children
B usually presents with visual failure
C causes hypothalamic abnormalities
D is diagnosed on skull X-ray
E prognosis is better than for pituitary adenoma

300. **Visual findings typical of hysteria include:**

A symmetrical field constriction
B tubular field on tangent screen testing
C central scotoma
D homonymous hemianopia
E optokinetic response on testing with an optokinetic drum

ANSWERS

Embryology and Anatomy

1. A   F   arises from the outer layer of the optic cup, which is neuroectoderm
    B   T
    C   T
    D   F   neuroectoderm
    E   T

2. A   F   ventral midbrain
    B   T
    C   F   ventral
    D   F   ventral
    E   F   ventral

3. A   T
    B   T
    C   T
    D   F   inferior oblique
    E   F   inferior oblique

4. A   T
    B   T
    C   F   contains fibres from motor root supplying the muscles of mastication
    D   T   leaves the skull through the foramen rotundum, then passes through the pterygopalatine fossa to the inferior orbital fissure
    E   F   the Gasserian ganglion occupies Meckel's cave, a recess in the petrous part of the temporal bone – it contains cells of origin of the trigeminal sensory axons. Cell bodies of the neurons innervating the muscles of mastication are found in the trigeminal mesencephalic nucleus

5. A   F   passes through foramen rotundum
    B   T
    C   T
    D   F   passes through foramen spinosum
    E   T

6. A T is an exocrine gland and produces a serous secretion
    B T and acinar cells
    C F parasympathetic is secretomotor, sympathetic is
          vasomotor
    D F sphenopalatine ganglion
    E F carries preganglionic fibres responsible for lacrimal
          secretion to the sphenopalatine ganglion where they
          synapse with postganglionic secretomotor neurons

7. A T because the posterior surface is more curved than the
          anterior surface
    B F 0.56 mm
    C T
    D T consists of collagen fibrils
    E F 90%

8. A F it lengthens to accommodate growth of the orbit
    B F optic stalk
    C F oligodendrocytes
    D T but can be congenitally myelinated
    E T

9. A T
    B F temporal to a vertical line through the fovea
    C F part of the thalamus
    D F alternating layers of grey and white matter
    E T

10. A F third ventricle
    B F paraventricular nucleus of hypothalamus
    C F supraoptic nucleus of hypothalamus
    D F hypothalamus
    E T

11. A T orbital plate of zygomatic bone
    B T
    C T
    D F constituent of the orbital roof
    E F the *nasolacrimal canal* is formed in the orbital aspect
          of the maxilla; the *lacrimal fossa* is formed between
          the frontal process of the maxilla and the lacrimal
          bone

12.	A	F	level of inferior colliculus (oculomotor nucleus is at level of superior colliculus)
	B	T	it is the only motor cranial nerve to do so
	C	F	the abducens nerve does
	D	F	it is the only motor cranial nerve to decussate
	E	F	it enters the orbit through the superior orbital fissure outside the annulus of Zinn, and remains outside the cone

13.	A	F	the outer layer of the optic cup develops into RPE; the inner, invaginated layer develops into neurosensory retina
	B	T	
	C	F	commences at the middle region of the cup (equator of the globe)
	D	T	melanisation is complete by the seventh week
	E	T	begins with bulging of nuclei in the ganglion cell layers, and is not complete until after birth

14.	A	F	ectoderm
	B	F	the first nucleus formed is the embryonic nucleus
	C	T	
	D	T	
	E	T	rubella virus particles have been isolated

15.	A	T	and endothelium
	B	T	
	C	F	neuroectoderm
	D	T	
	E	F	surface ectoderm

16.	A	T	because of the shorter distance from disc to nasal ora; retinopathy of prematurity initially affects the temporal periphery
	B	T	
	C	F	blood flow ceases in the seventh month and the artery disappears in the eighth
	D	T	
	E	T	

Physiology

17. A   T
    B   T
    C   T   rapid eye movement sleep
    D   F
    E   F   range = 30–700 degrees/sec

18. A   T
    B   T
    C   F   frontal cortex
    D   T   upward vertical saccades
    E   T

19. A   F   pursuit = 130 msec, saccade = 200–250 msec
    B   F
    C   F
    D   T
    E   T

20. A   F   parasympathetic
    B   T
    C   F   11D at 20 years, 15D at 4 years of age
    D   F
    E   F   normal AC/A ratio = 4 prism dioptres

21. A   F   it is more rapid in cones. The rapid first phase in the dark-adaptation curve represents the increase in sensitivity of the cones in the dark. This causes a typical 'kink' in the curve between five and ten minutes
    B   F   more sensitive to blue light (due to the Purkinje shift)
    C   T   liver and other stores of vitamin A must be exhausted before retinal effects become apparent
    D   F   full dark adaptation generally takes longer than 30 minutes
    E   T   this hereditary pigmentary retinopathy is caused by a disorder of phytanic acid metabolism. Retinitis pigmentosa also causes night blindness

22. A F 5–10μl
    B T
    C F IgG concentration is equal
    D T
    E F the mucin layer, contributed by conjunctiva, is deficient

23. A F most from aqueous, only 10% from tear film and limbal capillaries
    B T
    C T
    D T because it is fixed at the limbus
    E F

24. A T
    B T
    C F higher in late morning
    D T
    E F osmotic agents such as mannitol, which increase blood osmolarity, are used in therapy

25. A F 3.9 ml
    B T a component of vitrectomy irrigating solutions
    C F sodium hyaluronate, a mucopolysaccharide
    D F 98–99%
    E T but in a phakic subject these same wavelengths are absorbed by the lens

26. A T
    B F 33% (higher than any other organ in the body)
    C F actively extruded from the lens
    D T 25 times higher
    E T causing a gradual increase of lens thickness

27. A T
    B F
    C F
    D T
    E F

28. A F liver
     B T
     C T benign intracranial hypertension
     D F
     E T enhanced excretion

29. A F 6 mm
     B F 120 million rods, 6 million cones
     C T
     D F inner
     E F function in colour vision at mesopic light levels

30. A F
     B T optic atrophy implies destruction of the nerve fibres
     C F they enter on the temporal aspect of the nerve
     D F there is reduction of stimulus intensity and image
           blur on the retina
     E T

31. A T
     B F Mueller cells
     C F thought to arise from RPE
     D T
     E F

32. A T
     B T the bulk of formation is by this means
     C T
     D T plasma = 7 g/dl, aqueous = 0.02 g/dl; there is a
           dramatic increase following breakdown of the
           blood–aqueous barrier
     E F 10–50 times higher than plasma

Pathology

33. A F
     B T
     C F
     D T
     E T the herpesvirus group consists of at least 80 viruses,
           very few of which commonly affect man

34. A F Touton giant cells, characterised by vacuolated
           cytoplasm outside the ring of nuclei
     B T
     C F in a foreign body giant cell, nuclei are randomly
           arranged and foreign body fragments may be seen
     D T sometimes foreign body giant cells
     E T

35. A T characteristic of allergic reactions
     B T
     C F seen in chronic inflammatory reactions
     D T
     E F produce immunoglobulin and are derived from
           B-lymphocytes

36. A T fungi stain pink
     B F used for *Chlamydia*
     C T fungi stain purple
     D T fungi stain black against a green background
     E F used for Mycobacteria

37. A F
     B T
     C T
     D F
     E F

38. A F may be mistaken for squamous cell carcinoma
     B F elderly patients
     C T in the dermal layer
     D T and filled with keratin
     E T

39. A T
     B T usually being preceded by solar keratosis or
           carcinoma *in situ*
     C T in contrast to basal cell carcinoma
     D F this indicates differentiation and a better prognosis
     E T in the stroma and underlying dermis

40. A T
    B T
    C F tufted superficial vessels on the plaque are typical
    D F
    E T

41. A T and usually symmetrical
    B T the principal pathological feature
    C F periodic acid-Schiff is used
    D T it stains the amyloid
    E F this occurs in macular dystrophy and stains with
          periodic acid-Schiff

42. A T
    B F *rhegmatogenous* retinal detachment typically
          precedes proliferative vitreoretinopathy (PVR) – the
          latter may cause *traction* detachment
    C T and *epi*retinal membrane
    D T
    E F unless PVR is mild

43. A T intraocular calcification is uncommon in any other
          childhood condition
    B F rosettes indicate partial differentiation towards
          photoreceptors
    C F
    D F
    E F optic nerve invasion is of greater prognostic
          importance

44. A F 15 times commoner in whites
    B F
    C T
    D T
    E F *mixed cell* tumours, composed of a combination of
          spindle and epithelioid cells, are the commonest

45. A F via short posterior ciliary arteries to the choroid
    B T unlike choroidal melanoma
    C F such spread is rare
    D T
    E F

46. A F 50% of all lacrimal gland tumours consist of inflammatory and lymphoid proliferations, 25% are benign mixed tumours and 25% are adenoid cystic carcinomas
    B T a condensation of connective tissue
    C T these tumours must be excised *en bloc*, preserving the capsule to avoid tumour cell spread
    D T
    E F unlike patients with benign mixed tumours, these patients typically have pain due to tumour invasion along nerves

47. A F
    B T
    C F this occurs in children, usually aged less than 3 years
    D T usually proptosis of abrupt onset, or with Horner's syndrome or opsoclonus
    E T

48. A T nerve fibre layer defects are visible on ophthalmoscopy
    B F
    C T
    D T displaced posteriorly
    E T

49. A T *Chlamydia*
    B T *Neisseria gonorrhoeae*
    C T herpes simplex
    D T useful for gonococcus isolation (but not as useful as with genito-urinary infections)
    E F used in culture of Mycobacteria

50. A F this is the origin of primary optic nerve meningioma; arachnoid hyperplasia does occur
    B T
    C T may simulate meningioma
    D F this is the typical presentation of primary optic nerve meningioma; optic nerve glioma presents with proptosis and visual loss
    E F children or young adults

51. A F Corynebacteria are Gram-positive bacilli, typically cigar-shaped and arranged in pairs with a V-configuration
    B T coagulase-negative staphylococci and species of *Micrococcus* are also common commensals
    C T *Corynebacterium diphtheriae* infection
    D F the commonest source of antigen is staphylococcus. Non-ocular tuberculous infection is also important
    E F characteristically sensitive to the same antibiotics as other Gram-positive organisms

52. A F serotypes A–C
    B T serotypes D–K
    C T serotypes D–K
    D T serotypes D–K
    E F serotypes L^1–L^3

Pharmacology

53. A F inhibits protein synthesis
    B F inhibits protein synthesis
    C F inhibit protein synthesis
    D T cephalosporins also inhibit cell wall synthesis
    E F inhibit folate production

54. A T
    B T
    C T
    D F *hypo*kalaemia
    E T

55. A T and distal convoluted tubule
    B F independent
    C T
    D F metabolic *acidosis*
    E T Stevens–Johnson syndrome may occur as acetazolamide is related to the sulphonamides

56. A   T
    B   T
    C   F   noradrenaline acts at most
    D   T   acts at all postganglionic parasympathetic nerve endings
    E   T   in intracapsular cataract extraction

57. A   T   mydriasis results from either sympathetic stimulation or parasympathetic blockade. The near point of accommodation given is normal for a 20-year-old and indicates that the parasympathetic stimulation to accommodation has not been blocked
    B   F   sympatholytic
    C   F   parasympathomimetic
    D   T   sympathomimetic
    E   F   parasympatholytic

58. A   T
    B   F
    C   T
    D   F   inactivates noradrenaline
    E   T

59. A   F   a polyene antifungal agent
    B   T
    C   F   it is a macrolide used in the treatment of *Toxoplasma* retinochoroiditis
    D   T
    E   F   methicillin and cloxacillin are penicillinase-resistant

60. A   F   cyclooxygenase converts arachidonic acid to prostaglandin G_2, and is inhibited by nonsteroidal anti-inflammatory drugs
    B   T   inhibition of this enzyme may reduce cataract formation in diabetes mellitus
    C   T   this reaction in the lens causes cataract, as dulcitol increases intralenticular osmotic pressure
    D   T   and converts tyrosine to DOPA
    E   F   this reaction is catalysed by galactose-1-phosphate uridyl transferase; galactose kinase converts galactose to galactose-1-phosphate

61. A F receptors supplied by postganglionic
parasympathetic nerves are responsive to *muscarine*
   B T in an Adie pupil, administration of 0.1% pilocarpine
causes miosis due to denervation hypersensitivity
   C F pilocarpine causes *myopia* and this effect may be
substantial in patients aged less than 50 years
   D T
   E T

62. A T an indirectly acting muscarinic agonist
   B T this anaesthetic induction agent cannot be
metabolised
   C T the mechanism for this is unknown
   D T an adverse effect seen only in adults
   E T cholinesterase inhibitors are insecticides

63. A T it may acutely expand the blood volume
   B F
   C T not absorbed from the gastrointestinal tract
   D F 20% solution
   E T

64. A T
   B T both vestibular and auditory toxicity are
dose-related
   C F it may be administered in low doses, with particular
attention to serum trough drug levels
   D T aminoglycosides impair neuromuscular
transmission
   E T provided it is used at the appropriate dilution

65. A T
   B F ointment only
   C T
   D T it is phosphorylated by thymidine kinase, produced
by the virus
   E F resistance to acyclovir has not yet been encountered
in corneal herpes simplex infection

66. A T at time of discontinuation
   B F used in therapy
   C T
   D T if in high doses
   E F causes optic neuritis

67. A T 'Ganda' is a combination of gnanethidine and adrenaline
    B T Stevens–Johnson syndrome
    C T
    D F
    E T Stevens–Johnson syndrome

68. A T defective colour vision may be an early indication of overdosage
    B T it causes maculopathy
    C F
    D F
    E T it causes toxic optic neuropathy, as does ethambutol

Statistics

69. A F
    B F standard deviation equals the square root of the variance
    C F 68% of observations lie within one standard deviation of the mean; 95% lie within two standard deviations of the mean
    D T standard deviation is a measure of the dispersal of a group of observations around the mean
    E T
                                                        .

70. A F a larger sample will yield a smaller standard error
    B F
    C F parametric data is normally distributed
    D T then, based on the critical value of t, the null hypothesis is accepted or rejected
    E T

71. A F equal to or greater than zero
    B T
    C T
    D T
    E F $p < 0.05$ (5%) is taken as significant

Genetics

72. A T if heterozygous, the mutant gene is opposed by the modifying effect of the normal gene on the X-chromosome
    B T
    C T a male transmits his only X-chromosome to each daughter
    D F *none* of his sons are affected; the father transmits his Y-chromosome and not his X-chromosome to each son
    E T and half of her daughters will be carriers

73. A F autosomal recessive
    B T
    C F X-linked dominant
    D T
    E T

74. A F autosomal dominant
    B T this is the most common form of anomalous trichromacy, in which there is a red–green defect. In anomalous trichromats the three photopigments are present, but one is anomalous
    C F *ocular* albinism may be X-linked
    D T
    E F not a hereditary condition

Optics

75. A F
    B T
    C F
    D T
    E F

76. A T Base-in prisms are used for exodeviations
    B F
    C F
    D T
    E F

77. A F
    B T
    C T
    D T   minus
    E F

78. A T
    B F
    C T
    D F
    E T

79. A F   cylindrical lenses
    B T
    C F
    D T
    E F   red image

80. A T
    B T
    C F
    D T
    E T

81. A F
    B T
    C F
    D T
    E T   spherical aberration is the main reason for this impairment of visual acuity

82. A T
    B F
    C T
    D T
    E F

83. A T
    B F
    C T
    D T
    E F   the axial length of the eye is normal; the refractive power is inadequate. Therefore 'refraction hypermetropia'

84. A F hypermetropic or myopic spherical errors of > 4D are
                not corrected to 6/6 with a pin hole
     B T
     C T
     D F 1.33
     E T

85. A F
     B T to minimise aberrations
     C T the exact multiple depends on the observer's pupil size
                and the aperture of the condensing lens, which
                together determine the field of view. The field of
                illumination depends on the *subject's* pupil size
     D F
     E F

86. A T
     B F 1.5 D
     C F
     D T
     E T

87. A F
     B T
     C F
     D F
     E T

88. A T
     B T Thus to focus at 25 cm only 1 D of accommodation is
                used
     C F 14 D
     D F 3 D of accommodation is needed
     E T

89. A F
     B T
     C T
     D T
     E T

90. A   T
     B   T
     C   F   coherent
     D   F   monochromatic
     E   F   diffraction occurs at the pupil margin

91. A   F   1.33
     B   T   1.38
     C   T   1.41 } the refractive index of the cornea is 1.37
     D   F   1.33
     E   T   1.52

92. A   F   reflected *away from* the principal focus
     B   T
     C   F   second principal focus
     D   T
     E   F   light in the meridian parallel to the axis of a cylinder
             passes through undeviated. In the meridian at right
             angles to the axis, the cylinder acts as a spherical lens

93. A   F
     B   T
     C   F
     D   T
     E   T

94. A   F   basic plastic is poly(HEMA); PMMA is used in hard
             lenses
     B   F   widely used
     C   T
     D   T   hard lenses are more suitable if astigmatism exceeds
             1D
     E   F   a favourable indication

95. A   T   if there is chronic hypoxia
     B   T   due to reduced oxygen availability to epithelium
     C   F   most glucose comes from the aqueous humour
     D   T   demonstrable on endothelial specular microscopy
     E   F

96. A T there is a greater opportunity for heat to be conducted away from the smaller spot
    B F blue is 488 nm, green is 514.5 nm
    C F green is not absorbed by xanthophyll, but blue is absorbed and so is theoretically undesirable in photocoagulation of the posterior pole
    D T therefore less risk of nerve fibre layer damage
    E F less power: they induce less ocular scatter and have better penetration to the posterior segment

Lids and lacrimal apparatus

97. A T
    B T
    C F mild cases are very common in infants and resolve with age
    D T
    E T applied below the lashes, this may temporarily correct upward movement of preseptal orbicularis oculi

98. A T particularly in cicatricial ectropion, as the protective effect of Bell's phenomenon may be lost
    B F acute spastic *entropion* follows surgery
    C T congenital lower lid ectropion occurs
    D F ptosis is associated
    E T

99. A F visual incapacitation is usual
    B F nearly always bilateral
    C T muscles of forehead and cheek
    D F unlike hemifacial spasm
    E T for at least 6–8 weeks following injection

100. A F autosomal dominant, and some sporadic cases
     B F
     C T
     D T
     E T

101. A   T
      B   F   cardiac conduction defects would suggest dystrophia myotonica or Kearns–Sayre syndrome

      C   T
      D   T   pupil abnormalities are more likely to be caused by neurological diseases, such as Horner's syndrome or third cranial nerve palsy, than by muscle diseases

      E   F   no significant family history is noted in myasthenia gravis, other than in the neonatal variant

102. A   T
      B   F   it is due to synkinesis between levator palpebrae superioris, supplied by the oculomotor nerve, and the pterygoid, supplied by the trigeminal nerve

      C   T   surgical procedure is based on levator function. Many patients require a brow suspension

      D   T
      E   T

103. A   F   this operation is suitable if levator function exceeds 10 mm. For levator function between 5 and 10 mm, levator resection is appropriate

      B   T   for example in Horner's syndrome
      C   T   and the upper border of the tarsal plate and conjunctiva

      D   F   this complication is seen in large levator resections
      E   T   caused by the tarso-conjunctival suture

104. A   T   at least 4 mm
      B   F   perform these through the skin (anterior approach)
      C   F   for 5 mm of levator function, resect 22–26 mm of muscle; for 8–9 mm of levator function, resect 15 mm

      D   F   voluntary movement of levator aids in identification of lid structures

      E   F   this suture is placed in the lower lid

105. A   F
      B   T
      C   F
      D   F
      E   F   the typical improvement of a hypersensitivity reaction to staphylococcal exotoxins

106. A F a tumour >4 mm from the lid margin may require only a partial thickness excision
     B T
     C F they infiltrate deeply and are difficult to eradicate
     D F it may also arise from the glands of Zeis and sebaceous glands of the caruncle
     E T basal cell carcinoma accounts for >90%

107. A F children
     B F caused by a member of the poxvirus group
     C T they may have central umbilication and be multiple
     D F a chronic follicular conjunctival reaction is secondary to shedding of debris into the tear film
     E T

108. A T
     B T
     C T if total obstruction is present, dye testing is of no value
     D T this test result implies partial obstruction in the upper drainage system (at punctum, canaliculus or common canaliculus) or a defective lacrimal pump
     E F

109. A F this is a proliferation of basal cells in the epithelium
     B T occasionally progresses to squamous cell carcinoma
     C T occasionally progresses to squamous cell carcinoma
     D F
     E F

110. A F canaliculi remain patent
     B T
     C T and other causes of cicatrising conjunctivitis
     D T
     E F canaliculi remain patent

111. A F irrigation or probing should be avoided until infection subsides
     B T this will suffice if infection is not severe
     C T if severe infection
     D F DCR should be postponed until inflammation has subsided
     E T

Orbit

112. A F 15% of patients presenting with ocular signs are
              completely normal
      B T a feature of hypo- or hyperthyroidism
      C F it is the commonest cause of *axial* proptosis
      D F associated with pretibial myxoedema
      E T thyroid acropachy

113. A T
      B T
      C F more common in the elderly
      D F in childhood, rapidly growing primary tumours are
              more typically seen than secondary deposits.
              Neuroblastoma and acute leukaemia are two
              exceptions
      E F

114. A T
      B F slowly progressive axial proptosis
      C F young adult and middle-aged patients
      D F within the cone, usually inferior or lateral to the
              optic nerve
      E F diagnosed on CT scan, in which it enhances on
              contrast injection; also characteristically high
              amplitude internal echoes on A-scan ultrasound

115. A F young adult
      B F non-pulsatile proptosis, but it varies with central
              venous pressure (demonstrable by Valsalva's
              manoeuvre)
      C F uncommon
      D T
      E F this is the treatment of capillary haemangioma

116. A T or signs affecting the contralateral eye
      B T this vein is the major outflow of the cavernous sinus
      C T
      D T even ophthalmic artery occlusion
      E T and central retinal vein occlusion

117.
A T
B F age 20–40 years
C T
D T
E T usually dramatic improvement

118.
A T
B F this tumour is usually situated supranasally but may involve any part of the orbit
C T in the past, these tumours were treated by exenteration. Multidisciplinary treatment now comprises local irradiation and pulsed chemotherapy with vincristine, adriamycin and cyclophosphamide
D F biopsy is performed early for histopathological confirmation and pretreatment staging
E F presentation is usually painless but otherwise similar to orbital cellulitis

119.
A F by definition this is a fracture occurring in the floor or medial wall, independent of fracture of the orbital rim or adjacent facial bones
B T the fracture may be regarded as "protective"
C T
D F mydriasis may occur due to (a) damage to the parasympathetic pupillomotor fibres in the nerve to inferior oblique; or (b) traumatic mydriasis
E T

120.
A T mean age 45–50 years
B T unlike adenoid cystic carcinoma
C F
D F
E F the tumour should be removed with its capsule intact: if this is ruptured, the tumour becomes much more invasive

121.
A T ampicillin is suitable for *Haemophilus influenzae*, a common causative organism in children
B T cloxacillin is suitable for penicillinase-producing *Staphylococcus aureus*
C T confirm on CT scan and drain without delay
D F cavernous sinus thrombosis would cause rapid progression of proptosis and neurological signs
E T typically ketoacidotic diabetics

122.
A   F   it manifests primarily in the first year, often in the
          neonatal period
B   T   unlike a port wine stain
C   T   involutes spontaneously in the majority
D   T
E   F   unlike cavernous haemangioma

123.
A   T
B   F   this approach should be avoided if possible because
          of disturbance of later bone growth
C   T   and usually the orbital floor
D   F   Le Fort I: no orbital involvement
          Le Fort II: medial orbital floors involved
          Le Fort III: craniofacial dysjunction involving orbital
          floor and medial and lateral walls
E   F   not necessary unless the muscle is entrapped

124.
A   F   only if there is diplopia in primary position and/or
          downgaze
B   F
C   T   especially if cosmetically unacceptable
D   F   this indicates probable orbital haemorrhage and
          possible optic nerve damage, and is not an indication
          for surgery at the time most patients present
E   F   a common finding that usually improves

125.
A   T   used early in the management of optic nerve
          compression, radiotherapy may diminish the
          requirement for steroids
B   F   strabismus often increases, with a tendency to
          esotropia and hypotropia
C   T   since muscle balance is dynamic and, as a general rule,
          strabismus surgery is performed if deviation is stable
          for more than six months
D   T   advisable in every case for the same reason
E   F   increased proptosis is seen in the event of large
          recessions of inferior and medial recti

126.
A   T
B   F   displacement is axial, unless there is a subperiosteal
          abscess
C   T   particularly in children
D   T
E   F   children usually respond to treatment without
          complications. Adults more frequently develop
          complications such as intracranial infection

Conjunctiva and cornea

127. A F
      B T
      C T infants with aniridia and cystinosis are highly photophobic
      D F
      E T patients with this infection have pain and photophobia which is usually more severe than the clinical signs suggest

128. A T
      B T
      C T
      D T a patient with translocation Down's syndrome has trisomy 21, but only 46 chromosomes, as the extra chromosome 21 is translocated to a D group chromosome (usually chromosome 14). The risk is less than expected, approx. 10% instead of 33%, because most Down's conceptuses are aborted. 95% of cases of Down's syndrome are due to nondisjunction rather than translocation, resulting in 47 chromosomes. The parents of these cases are genetically normal, and the risk of recurrence in a sibling (maternal age < 37 years) is 1–2% (cf. 1:600 for general population)
      E F this is Edwards' syndrome

129. A F usually bilateral although sometimes asymmetrical
      B F epithelium usually intact
      C T
      D T unlike Mooren's ulcer
      E F most often males over 60 years

130. A F lymphocytic response
      B T
      C T
      D T
      E F mixed polymorph and lymphocytic response

131. A T
     B T tarsal follicles and Gram-negative diplobacilli on
          smear
     C T
     D T
     E F papillary hypertrophy

132. A T
     B T
     C T
     D T
     E F subhyaloid or *vitreous* haemorrhage is associated

133. A T
     B T also adenovirus
     C T also β-haemolytic streptococci and
          Corynebacterium diphtheriae
     D F
     E T marked thickening of the upper tarsal conjunctiva
          occurs in this condition

134. A T also contact lens wear
     B T the papillae are polygonal ("cobblestones") and
          have a flat surface
     C F *Acanthamoeba* causes keratitis only
     D F a follicular reaction is usual in preservative toxicity
          and adenovirus infection
     E F

135. A T
     B T
     C F
     D F *herpes simplex* causes pannus formation, usually
          >2 mm
     E T

136. A F
     B T
     C T
     D F
     E T

137. A T
     B T herpes zoster is the most frequent local cause of
          scleritis
     C F this is seen in stromal infection by herpes simplex,
          Acanthamoeba and fungi
     D T entropion may occur due to lid scarring; ectropion,
          trichiasis and ptosis may also occur
     E T

138. A F distribution is subepithelial and in the anterior part
          of Bowman's layer
     B T
     C T
     D T the cornea is a site of ectopic calcification caused by
          the hypercalcaemia occurring in renal failure
     E F band keratopathy may be cleared by removal of
          overlying epithelium and EDTA application, or by
          excimer laser

139. A F
     B F
     C T
     D F
     E T also in microcystic and macular dystrophies

140. A T irregular astigmatism and axial myopia
     B F very rare
     C T
     D T however, the patient may require further contact lens
          correction for surgically induced astigmatism
     E T as are other atopic disorders such as eczema

141. A F more prevalent and severe in males
     B F ultraviolet
     C F
     D T there is opacification or elevation of the central area
          of capsule exposed by the undilated pupil
     E T also affects Bowman's layer

142. A T
     B T
     C F
     D F there is a higher risk of allograft rejection due to
          vascularisation
     E F

143. A   T   also, less commonly, enteroviruses, coxsackieviruses and adenoviruses

     B   F

     C   F   but the condition is self-limiting

     D   T   although corneal ulcers have occurred in some patients in some epidemics

     E   F   discomfort and lacrimation are common

144. A   F   it is caused by *Chlamydia trachomatis*, serotypes D-K

     B   T

     C   T

     D   F

     E   F   treated with topical and systemic tetracycline

145. A   F   trachoma is typically found in dry, dusty climates, and prevalence is proportional to distance from water supply

     B   T

     C   T

     D   F   no vaccine is yet available

     E   F   the Giemsa stain is useless in trachoma, although helpful in neonatal and adult inclusion conjunctivitis. The diagnosis is essentially clinical. Culture from conjunctival swabs is useful in research but impractical

146. A   T

     B   T

     C   T   occlusion therapy for amblyopia may be necessary

     D   F   lens wear is associated with giant papillary conjunctivitis

     E   T   and atopes

147. A   F   conjunctival scarring secondary to trachoma or bacterial infection is commonest

     B   F   several topical glaucoma medications have been more commonly implicated. Practolol has been withdrawn from use, except for intravenous administration in acute cardiac arrhythmias

     C   T

     D   T   due to symblepharon and loss of fornix

     E   F   there is frequent recurrence, particularly in ocular cicatricial pemphigoid

148.   A   F   pseudopterygium occurs
       B   F   although a pathological feature is destruction of Bowman's layer by fibroblasts
       C   T   due to growth across the central cornea
       D   T   especially after repeated excisions
       E   F

149.   A   T   if refractory to other treatments
       B   F   visualisation of the cornea and anterior chamber are immediately reduced by the flap
       C   T   slight ptosis is common, resulting from conjunctival dissection at the superior fornix
       D   F   perforation of the flap at surgery is a major complication, but flap retraction is very common
       E   T   other alternatives are protective ptosis induced by botulinum toxin, and cyanoacrylate blepharorrhaphy.

150.   A   T
       B   F
       C   T   colobomas of the upper eyelid are common in Goldenhar's syndrome, a component of which is epibulbar dermoid
       D   F   Goldenhar's syndrome is congenital and not hereditary
       E   T

151.   A   F   unlike acne vulgaris
       B   T
       C   T
       D   T   improves skin and ocular manifestations
       E   T

152.   A   F   no malignant potential
       B   F   rarely
       C   T   formerly called precancerous melanosis, malignant change eventually occurs in 20-30% of these patients. This is suggested by nodularity, which implies that the lesion is invasive
       D   F   this is seen in pregnancy and Addison's disease
       E   F

153. A   T   partial or complete biopsy of suspicious lesions
      B   T   for intraocular spread
      C   T   for orbital spread
      D   T   may be combined with local excision
      E   F

Glaucoma

154. A   T   a potential problem in cataract surgery
      B   F   *hyper*pigmentation
      C   T
      D   T   another potential problem in cataract surgery
      E   T   60% of eyes affected by pseudoexfoliation

155. A   F   increases
      B   T
      C   T
      D   F   there is a lack of pigmentation, all angle structures
                having a 'washed out' appearance
      E   F

156. A   F   cup symmetry is usual in non-glaucoma patients
      B   T   an important sign for progression of field loss
      C   F
      D   T
      E   T

157. A   F   the trabecular meshwork stretches from Schwalbe's
                line to the scleral spur
      B   T
      C   T   prior to puberty
      D   F   occasionally visible if the trabecular meshwork has
                little pigmentation
      E   F

158. A   T   ferry line anterior to the filtration bleb
      B   T   'malignant' glaucoma is due to aqueous misdirection
      C   T
      D   F
      E   T

159. A F
      B T four times as common as OAG in one survey in Burma
      C T if chronic angle-closure glaucoma
      D T if chronic angle-closure glaucoma
      E T a reason for visual loss in an acute attack

160. A F this causes raised intra*cranial* pressure
      B F
      C T
      D T
      E T

161. A F reduced
      B T there is marked hypermetropia
      C F secondary angle-closure glaucoma
      D F it is abnormally *thick*, and may impede vortex venous drainage
      E T choroidal effusion and non-rhegmatogenous retinal detachment frequently complicate intraocular surgery

162. A T
      B T less commonly than *central* retinal vein occlusion
      C F
      D F *proliferative* diabetic retinopathy
      E T

163. A F undertake panretinal photocoagulation if the media are clear, or peripheral retinal cryotherapy if not
      B T this may be successful in early cases
      C T there will be a higher chance of success if laser can regress the new vessels and thus prevent their growth into the filtering bleb
      D F topical steroid and atropine will make the eye more comfortable; otherwise a cycloablative procedure can be performed. Evisceration is the last option
      E T

164. A F intermittent *open*-angle glaucoma
      B T due to forward displacement of the iris–lens diaphragm
      C T
      D F glaucoma may develop years after injury
      E T treated by lens extraction

165. A F
     B F both features of mesodermal dysgenesis (Axenfeld's and Rieger's anomalies)
     C T
     D F glaucoma is secondary to corneal endothelial overgrowth in the anterior chamber, and formation of peripheral anterior synechiae
     E F young adult life or middle age

166. A F bilateral in 65–75%, but frequently asymmetrical
     B T Haab's striae
     C F the cupping may regress if IOP is normalised
     D T management is essentially surgical
     E F abnormal findings include Barkan's membrane extending from Schwalbe's line over the angle, and peripheral iris stromal hypoplasia

167. A T and secondary nystagmus
     B T
     C F Wilms' tumour occurs in the sporadic cases; deletion of the short arm of chromosome 11 is found in some
     D T exclude the tumour by ultrasound or intravenous urography in infants with aniridia
     E T 50% develop glaucoma

168. A F autosomal dominant
     B T
     C F
     D F
     E T

Lens

169. A T assuming the patient is alert and cooperative. Loss of light perception should never be explained on the basis of cataract alone
     B T however, confident light projection in some quadrants but not others suggests posterior segment problems such as branch retinal vein or artery occlusion, partial retinal detachment, or a dependent vitreous haemorrhage
     C F this finding must prompt a search for other ocular abnormalities
     D F testing for light perception or hand movements in field quadrants may be informative in the presence of significant lens opacities
     E F B-scan ultrasound should be performed in eyes with mature cataract

170. A   F   causes cornea verticillata and maculopathy
     B   T   used in chronic myeloid leukaemia
     C   F   caused by hypoparathyroidism and conditions
               giving rise to hypocalcaemia
     D   F   dystrophia myotonica gives rise to cataract
     E   T

171. A   T
     B   T
     C   T   resulting from contaminated irrigating solutions
     D   F   although iris trauma does occur
     E   T

172. A   T   intracapsular extraction is indicated
     B   F   the size of the lens nucleus determines section width.
               This is the same for extra- and endocapsular
               extraction methods
     C   F
     D   F   capsule is removed *after* lens insertion
     E   F   theoretically, endocapsular extraction protects the
               corneal endothelium

173. A   F
     B   T   particularly in young patients
     C   F
     D   T
     E   F

174. A   T
     B   F   most commonly it is an isolated finding; congenital
               cataract may be associated with microphthalmos or
               coloboma, and in a few patients is part of a systemic
               syndrome
     C   T   autosomal dominant inheritance is by far the most
               common mode of inheritance. Some cases are
               autosomal recessive or X-linked
     D   F   only a small percentage
     E   T

175. A T
    B F   a sunflower pattern cataract occurs due to copper deposition in the anterior subcapsular cortex
    C F   patients are often troubled by bright sunlight or car headlights even when visual acuity in a dark room is good
    D F   near acuity is affected first
    E T

176. A T   this is a long-acting cholinesterase inhibitor
    B T   if administered orally
    C F
    D T   seen in Fabry's disease
    E T   this is suggestive of retinitis pigmentosa, which is associated with cataract

177. A F
    B T
    C F   usually associated with ocular hypotony
    D T   this rare complication consists of downgrowth of conjunctival epithelium through a wound defect. Cells invade the trabecular network and cause intractable glaucoma
    E T   it causes uveitis and secondary glaucoma

178. A F   *S.epidermidis*
    B T   *Propionobacterium acnes* causes low-grade late endophthalmitis
    C T   usually gradual onset and presents about one week postoperatively
    D F   starch from surgical gloves causes severe uveitis, which presents two to eight days postoperatively and responds to steroid
    E T

179. A T
    B T
    C F   posterior chamber lens implantation is contraindicated only if the zonule is involved and cannot support a posterior chamber lens. In that event, an anterior chamber lens would be more suitable
    D F   depending on the extent and site of the tear, it may be safe to proceed
    E T   however, YAG laser is increasingly used in place of primary surgical capsulotomy

180. A F this is gyrate atrophy, in which condition the lens is normal
     B T
     C T
     D T also Marfan's syndrome and homocystinuria
     E F

181. A T sphincterotomy may be necessary to allow nucleus expression
     B F
     C F
     D T
     E F although open angle glaucoma is associated

182. A F maximal at two to four hours
     B F pits and cracks rarely cause glare
     C F this complication may rarely complicate surgical capsulotomy
     D T
     E F it is considered wise to wait until at least six months following surgery to reduce the risk of cystoid macular oedema

183. A T also causes true exfoliation of the lens capsule, seen in glass blowers
     B T lens opacity is associated with climatic keratopathy
     C T
     D F
     E T

Uveal tract

184. A T congenital Horner's syndrome
     B T
     C F
     D F
     E T siderosis

185. A F arthritis confined to four joints or less at presentation is termed *pauci*articular, and is associated with uveitis
B F the child typically presents to the eye clinic with visual loss from band keratopathy, glaucoma or cataract in a *white* eye
C F
D T
E F band keratopathy

186. A T
B F 70–96% reported
C F
D F follicular
E F most patients return to normal health

187. A F 10–20%
B F >90%
C F it is a seronegative arthropathy
D F conjunctivitis is a feature of Reiter's syndrome
E F sacro-iliac joints

188. A T bilateral diffuse granulomatous uveitis
B T unlike sympathetic ophthalmia, and leads to a chorioretinal scar
C T vitiligo
D F these are seen in juvenile xanthogranuloma
E T

189. A T
B T
C T
D F skin signs include keratoderma blenorrhagica and circinate balanitis
E T

190. A T
B T
C T these could represent choroidal tubercles, seen in miliary tuberculosis
D T in addition to tuberculous optic nerve infiltration, neuropathy may follow ethambutol, isoniazid or streptomycin therapy
E T

191.   A   F   keratic precipitates are diffusely scattered but do *not* pigment
      B   F   no mydriatic is necessary
      C   T   evident on flourescein angiography
      D   T   secondary open-angle glaucoma in 20%
      E   F   one survey found disease to be bilateral in 11%

192.   A   T
      B   T
      C   T   cotton wool patches
      D   F
      E   T

193.   A   F   anterior uveitis is not a feature of POHS and if many cells are seen in the aqueous, this casts doubt on the diagnosis
      B   T   'histo spots'
      C   T   subretinal neovascular membranes give rise to permanent impairment of central acuity
      D   F
      E   F   intraocular candidiasis occurs in drug abusers

194.   A   F   an obligate *intra*cellular parasite
      B   F   spread in cat faeces
      C   F   intra*cerebral* calcification results from intrauterine infection
      D   F   a positive dye test indicates that the patient has had *Toxoplasma* infection at some time in the past. Theoretically, rising titres indicate recent infection. ELISA for specific IgM identifies recent infection
      E   T   300 mg four times daily (adult dose) if central vision is threatened

195.   A   T
      B   T
      C   T
      D   F   *anterior* uveitis
      E   F   pigmentary retinopathy may be acquired

196.	A	F	microfilariae cause inflammation when they die
	B	T	in the anterior chamber
	C	T	it has superseded diethylcarbamazine which caused a Mazzotti reaction with enhanced inflammation on treatment
	D	F	
	E	T	also conjunctivitis, keratitis, anterior and posterior uveitis

197.	A	T	20–30% of patients with systemic sarcoidosis have ocular inflammation
	B	F	periphlebitis
	C	F	*non*caseating
	D	F	a sarcoid granuloma of the optic nerve may occur
	E	F	this test is widely used. Intradermal injection of sarcoid spleen induces granuloma formation at 4–6 weeks in patients with sarcoidosis

198.	A	T	sectorial cataract in some patients
	B	T	rarely epithelioid
	C	T	indicated only in the diffuse type of melanoma
	D	F	iris melanomas constitute less than 10% of all uveal melanomas; ciliary body melanomas account for approximately 15%
	E	T	with the exception of the diffusely growing type, these tumours have 'benign' biological behaviour

199.	A	F	*S. epidermidis*
	B	T	this is typical although some cases present earlier. Bacterial infection is very much more common
	C	F	*Propionobacterium* endophthalmitis presents as late postoperative uveitis
	D	T	also chemosis: these signs are typical of infective and not sterile postoperative inflammation
	E	T	

200.	A	F	the tumour lethal dose for retinoblastoma is 40 Gy and for melanoma 60–100 Gy
	B	F	localised choroidal haemangioma and melanoma cause serous detachment
	C	T	liver is most common
	D	F	drugs are used in palliative therapy of metastatic disease only
	E	T	if the tumour thickness is 3 mm or less

201.

A	F	it arises from non-pigmented ciliary epithelium and is composed of cells resembling primitive medullary cells of the CNS
B	T	in young adults
C	F	
D	F	
E	T	

202.

A	T	both are features of Sturge–Weber syndrome. The meningeal angioma may give rise to Jacksonian epilepsy
B	F	
C	F	posterior pole
D	F	
E	F	laser is indicated if serous retinal detachment threatens the macula. The aim is to create a chorioretinal adhesion

203.

A	T	
B	F	bronchus
C	T	infiltrate laterally
D	F	choroidal metastases are nearly ten times as common
E	T	clinical response is observed at 4–6 weeks

Vitreous & retina

204.

A	T	
B	T	high altitude retinal haemorrhages are seen often in young healthy subjects
C	T	
D	T	papilloedema
E	T	severe retinopathy is seen with this form of sickle-cell disease

205.

A	F	unlike anterior scleritis
B	T	may be mistaken for a choroidal tumour
C	T	exudative retinal detachment
D	T	this demonstrates thickening of the sclera
E	F	high dose systemic steroid with or without other immunosuppressive agents are used

206.
A	T	
B	F	autosomal recessive
C	F	of the inherited forms, autosomal dominant is the most benign
D	T	subsequent to chronic cystoid macular oedema
E	T	and may involve the macula

207.
A	T	scotopic ERG is abnormal
B	T	the ERG is extinguished relatively early in disease, and has little use in monitoring progression
C	F	EOG light rise is absent
D	T	
E	F	

208.
A	F	this is Usher's syndrome; Refsum's syndrome includes pigmentary retinopathy, polyneuritis, cerebellar signs and electrocardiographic signs
B	T	given in very high doses, it has a beneficial effect on retinal and neurological signs
C	F	ERG
D	T	poorly understood
E	F	increased phytanic acid levels occur in Refsum's disease, due to deficiency of phytanic acid hydroxylase. Gyrate atrophy is associated with increased ornithine levels, due to deficiency of ornithine ketoacid aminotransferase

209.
A	F	X-linked
B	F	central vision is last to be affected
C	F	unlike retinitis pigmentosa
D	F	unlike retinitis pigmentosa
E	F	the ERG and EOG are markedly abnormal early in the disease

210.
A	F	EOG is abnormal long before visual acuity falls
B	T	
C	F	autosomal dominant with variable penetrance
D	F	EOG
E	T	EOG abnormalities in carriers

211. A   T   but production of melanin is greatly reduced due to diminished enzymatic oxidation of tyrosine
      B   T
      C   F   on account of abnormal decussation at the chiasm, each hemisphere receives predominantly monocular input from the contralateral eye. Therefore albinos lack the anatomical substrate for binocular single vision
      D   F   spherical and cylindrical errors are very common
      E   T   giant melanosomes are pathognomonic

212. A   T
      B   T
      C   F   6/9–6/12, and vision can be improved with a weak convex lens
      D   T   in non-arteritic ischaemic optic neuropathy, visual acuity is usually better
      E   T

213. A   F   these cause no problems, unlike holes posterior to the vitreous base
      B   T   this is likely to progress to retinal detachment
      C   F   risk of retinal detachment is very small
      D   T   this is similar to lattice degeneration with potential for break formation
      E   F   a frequent finding in normal eyes

214. A   T
      B   F   traction retinal detachment
      C   T
      D   T
      E   F   traction retinal detachment

215. A   F
      B   F   microphthalmos
      C   F   unilateral in 90%
      D   T   in anterior PHPV, they are elongated and easily visible
      E   F   these patients need removal of cataract and retrolental mass by closed intraocular microsurgery, correction of aphakia and treatment of amblyopia

216.
A	T	after panretinal photocoagulation
B	T	with a break in Bruch's membrane
C	T	
D	T	
E	T	this often follows iridotomy, and rarely follows panretinal photocoagulation when annular ciliochoroidal detachment arises. Anterior displacement of the iris–lens diaphragm may lead to angle-closure glaucoma

217.
A	T	panretinal photocoagulation may cause the neovascular process to regress, allowing successful filtration surgery
B	F	
C	T	
D	T	some patients respond well to grid macular photocoagulation
E	T	used in some patients. It shortens the duration of symptoms but does not improve visual prognosis

218.
A	T	
B	F	only mild ocular disease is seen, despite severe systemic manifestations
C	T	SC disease and SThal patients have severe ocular disease but mild systemic disease
D	T	pigmentary retinopathy, spinocerebellar atrophy, acanthocytosis and fat malabsorption occur
E	F	usually regresses

219.
A	T	vitreous traction
B	T	after initially being flat, vessels become elevated
C	T	particularly after encircling procedures
D	F	
E	T	due to ischaemia

220.
A	F	'dragged' disc is typical
B	F	retrolental mass occurs
C	T	
D	T	traction at the temporal periphery leads to a dragged disc and macular ectopia
E	F	

221.
A	F	between Bruch's membrane and the retinal pigment epithelium
B	T	if longstanding; this causes glistening
C	T	disc drüsen
D	T	disc drüsen
E	F	ERG is normal

222.
A	F	acuity should be better than 6/36, indicating location outside the foveal avascular zone
B	T	likely to be outside the foveal avascular zone
C	F	laser is contraindicated as the RPE may tear
D	T	
E	T	krypton and green-only argon laser do not harm the nerve fibre layer and therefore are considered to be better suited for macular photocoagulation. However, argon laser, either green-only or blue-green, is most frequently used

223.
A	T	this detachment is smaller than the serous retinal elevation and gives rise to a small hyperfluorescent spot early in fluorescein angiography
B	F	
C	T	
D	F	males, age 20–40 years
E	F	congenital optic disc pit is associated

224.
A	F	this retinopathy follows compression injury to the head or trunk
B	T	
C	F	
D	T	
E	F	cotton wool patches clear within weeks

225.
A	T	leakage occurs from blood vessels undergoing traction
B	T	
C	T	
D	T	it is dominantly inherited, and has an early onset followed by a protracted course
E	F	it is caused by retinitis pigmentosa

226. A   T   'cartwheel' maculopathy results from cystoid schitic changes within the foveola
     B   F   decreased scotopic B-wave amplitude is found
     C   T
     D   T   secondary to retinoschisis
     E   F

227. A   F   breaks occur in *Bruch's membrane* with secondary changes in the RPE
     B   T   due to RPE window defects
     C   T   causing loss of central vision
     D   F   Paget's disease, pseudoxanthoma elasticum, Ehlers–Danlos syndrome and sickle-cell disease
     E   T   non-ocular features of this syndrome are joint hyperextensibility and skin hyperelasticity

228. A   F
     B   T   the basis is thought to be vascular, with retinal arteriolar occlusion
     C   T
     D   T
     E   T   SSPE is a rare complication of measles causing pigmentary maculopathy and cortical blindness. EEG findings are diagnostic

229. A   T
     B   F   50% as the condition is autosomal dominant
     C   F   50%
     D   F   in one series, median age at diagnosis was 8 months for children with bilateral tumours and 25 months for those with unilateral tumours
     E   F   orbital spread precedes metastases, and bone metastases are commonest, characteristically under the scalp

230. A   T   80% of patients with tuberous sclerosis have epilepsy
     B   F   treatment is unnecessary
     C   F   it is associated with tuberous sclerosis. Sturge–Weber syndrome is associated with choroidal haemangioma
     D   T   typically periventricular astrocytic harmartomas in tuberous sclerosis
     E   T   similar to those seen in neurofibromatosis

231. A F only if proliferative vitreoretinopathy arises
      B T the most frequent indication
      C F
      D T
      E T

232. A T
      B F proliferative
      C T
      D F proliferative
      E F

233. A T
      B T
      C F the juvenile form is X-linked
      D F juvenile form
      E T surgery is rarely indicated

Motility

234. A T
      B F the opposite is true
      C F bilateral lateral rectus resection is indicated
      D T
      E T conjunctiva may be recessed to the original muscle
            insertion

235. A F
      B T it is thicker than in adults and is not adherent to
            bulbar conjunctiva
      C F no limitation follows resection of less than 8 mm of
            lateral rectus
      D F
      E T through a limbal conjunctival incision

236.
A F   the maximum recession necessary is initially performed so that adjustment will involve readvancement

B T

C F   the patient must be able to cooperate for suture adjustment

D F   it is particularly suited to mechanical limitations of this type, with frequent involvement of vertical muscles and diplopia

E F   it is suitable for consecutive exotropia and cosmetic operations in older patients with a risk of postoperative diplopia

237.
A T

B T   the test subtends (on the macula) 6° for near and 1.5° for distance. A microtrope fuses for near and not distance

C T

D T   this is diplopia

E F   alternating suppression must be occurring

238.
A F   secondary actions of vertical recti are adduction and of obliques are abduction

B T

C F

D T

E F

239.
A F

B T   by dissociating the eyes for near vision

C T   and horizontal

D F   binocular single vision is needed for a normal result in this test

E F   upshoot implies a superior oblique palsy

240.
A F   in contrast to older children with accommodative esotropia

B T

C T

D T

E F   these children do not develop amblyopia. Occlusion is however useful in differential diagnosis of sixth cranial nerve palsy

241. A T however, these patients have binocularity on the basis of peripheral fusion
    B T
    C F variable, 6/9–6/60
    D T confirmed by the 4 dioptre prism test
    E T

242. A T
    B F tests fusion
    C T
    D F tests fusion
    E F tests simultaneous perception and fusion

243. A F normal
    B F rare
    C T provided they are well fitted
    D T it allows sufficient accommodation to take place for clear vision without associated convergence
    E T either bimedial recession or a Faden procedure to both medial recti

244. A F a progressive weakening is produced as the eye moves into the field of action of the muscle
    B T
    C T
    D T the superior rectus is sutured
    E F the technique is usually used in lateral rectus palsy, in which the suture is applied to the contralateral synergist of the paralysed muscle. This results in greater concomitance

245. A F V-pattern
    B F incomitant
    C F a minor increase in the horizontal deviation is seen in most patients
    D T although often asymmetrical, bilateral surgery is usually performed
    E T or recession

246. A T
    B T
    C T convergence deteriorates late
    D T patients stimulate convergence by inducing accommodation
    E F

247. A F   usually unilateral and affecting the left side most commonly
      B T   a rare symptom
      C F   BSV is maintained by an abnormal head posture
      D T
      E F   only if abnormal head posture or noticeable deviation in primary position result in poor cosmesis

248. A F   lower field
      B F   *inferior* oblique palsy is simulated
      C T
      D F   spontaneous improvement occurs
      E F   this is very slight, unlike in inferior oblique palsy

Neuro-ophthalmology

249. A T
      B T
      C T
      D F
      E F

250. A T
      B F   if a pupil abnormality is suspected, it is important to test the reactions in light and dark
      C F   cocaine is used in the confirmation of a defect of the sympathetic pathway, which causes a constricted pupil
      D T   0.1% pilocarpine drops are used in the diagnosis of an Adie pupil. This dilute concentration causes pupil constriction in the phase of denervation hypersensitivity
      E F   used in differentiation of pre- and postganglionic Horner's syndrome

251. A F   the consensual reflex is normal
      B T
      C T
      D T   lesions in any part of the anterior visual pathway cause an afferent defect
      E F   pupil reactions are normal in a cortical lesion

252.

A	T
B	T	the sympathetic nerves are a constituent of the lumen of the cavernous sinus (also the sixth cranial nerve and the internal carotid artery). Accordingly, Horner's syndrome would be expected as an early sign in any sinus lesion
C	T	particularly thyroid carcinoma with local spread
D	T	
E	T	

253.

A	T
B	F	this pupil 'accommodates but does not react'
C	F	
D	T	
E	F	

254.

A	T	usually hemianopic 'band' optic atrophy
B	F	
C	T	described as 'waxy' pallor
D	T	
E	T	optic nerve glioma is a recognised and important feature of neurofibromatosis

255.

A	T	infants have head nodding
B	F	it occurs in the first two years of life
C	F	
D	T	uniocular nystagmus
E	F	

256.

A	T	'ataxic' horizontal nystagmus is seen in the abducting eye
B	T	latent nystagmus is seen only in the eye under cover
C	F	binocular
D	F	binocular
E	T	

257.

A	F	downbeat nystagmus is seen in foramen magnum lesions
B	F	
C	T	particularly phenytoin
D	T	also horizontal jerk nystagmus
E	F	convergence–retraction nystagmus can be elicited

258. A F it is situated in the midbrain ventral to the aqueduct
      B T in a lesion of the third cranial nerve nucleus, contralateral superior rectus weakness and bilateral ptosis occur. These findings correspond with the organisation of the subnuclei
      C T
      D T a small degree of proptosis can be measured
      E T transient third cranial nerve palsy occurs in ophthalmoplegic migraine. Permanent signs may follow repeated episodes

259. A F
      B F
      C T chronic middle ear and mastoid infection cause osteitis of the petrous temporal bone leading to sixth cranial nerve palsy (Gradenigo's syndrome). The paralysis of abduction is associated with ipsilateral facial pain and deafness
      D T
      E T self-limiting sixth cranial nerve palsy is frequently associated with an exanthematous viral illness in childhood

260. A T due to an orbital apex inflammatory mass
      B T due to fifth cranial nerve involvement
      C F usually an early and beneficial response is seen
      D F CT scan
      E T due to involvement of cranial nerves at the orbital apex

261. A F most patients are asymptomatic
      B F the vergence centre is in the midbrain and not involved in a classical medial longitudinal bundle lesion
      C T especially if bilateral
      D T in the abducting eye
      E F

262. A   F
     B   T   the horizontal gaze centre is in the parapontine reticular formation, adjacent to the sixth cranial nerve nucleus
     C   F
     D   F   because the vergence centre is in the midbrain
     E   F   a vascular lesion would be more likely. In young adults and children, demyelination and intrinsic brainstem glioma would respectively be the most likely causes

263. A   F   visual obscurations are typical
     B   T
     C   T   raised intracranial pressure may cause a sixth cranial nerve palsy
     D   T   it is essential to exclude an intracranial mass lesion, obstruction of ventricles or intracranial infection before making a diagnosis of benign intracranial hypertension
     E   T   the condition is self-limiting in many patients. However, treatment with acetazolamide, and, later, optic nerve sheath decompression, may be indicated if field loss occurs

264. A   T
     B   F
     C   T   the pyramidal tracts and seventh cranial nerve may be involved in a pontine lesion
     D   T
     E   T

265. A   T   tumours in this location are usually acoustic neuromas which cause cerebellar and fifth, seventh and eighth cranial nerve signs. A dry eye results because (a) the seventh cranial nerve is secretomotor to the lacrimal gland and (b) there is poor spreading of the tear film by the lids
     B   T
     C   T
     D   T
     E   F

266. A   F   partial ptosis
     B   T   as in thyroid disease
     C   T
     D   T   Collier's sign
     E   F

267. A   T   convergence–retraction nystagmus
     B   F   but there is near-light dissociation of pupil reactions
     C   T   saccadic vertical gaze is typically involved earlier in
                  disease than pursuit gaze
     D   F   the third cranial nerve nucleus is in the ventral
                  midbrain
     E   F   optic nerve is normal

268. A   F   seen in late 'vintage' papilloedema
     B   T   this is the only field abnormality
     C   T
     D   F
     E   F

269. A   T
     B   T
     C   F   optic neuritis causes a central scotoma. An
                  altitudinal defect is typical of anterior ischaemic
                  optic neuropathy
     D   T   for example, patients with demyelination are
                  frequently found to have delayed latency on VER in
                  the absence of any history of visual disturbance
     E   F

270. A   T
     B   F   cause disc swelling
     C   T
     D   T
     E   T

271. A   F
     B   T   saccadic paralysis
     C   F   this reflex is used by the patient to locate objects in
                  the visual environment
     D   F   in fact, infants with this disorder may be
                  misdiagnosed as blind
     E   T   characteristic

272.
A	F	seen with *dorsal* midbrain lesions
B	F	signs of pyramidal tract involvement are *contralateral*
C	T	indicates red nucleus involvement
D	T	
E	T	aneurysm of the posterior communicating artery in the interpeduncular region causes a widely dilated pupil

273.
A	F	these are intact
B	F	saccadic downgaze is lost first
C	T	after vertical gaze
D	T	
E	F	this condition affects the late middle-aged and elderly

274.
A	F	anterolateral to the aqueduct
B	T	
C	T	unlike third and sixth cranial nerve palsies
D	F	it usually follows closed head injuries, often in road traffic accidents
E	F	Brown's (superior oblique tendon sheath) syndrome is due to a restriction of superior oblique movement, not paralysis

275.
A	F	
B	F	this rapid and fine oscillation is seen in extreme gaze positions: it represents an abnormal strain on a normal gaze mechanism
C	T	this is a form of jerk nystagmus which undergoes cyclic changes in amplitude and direction
D	T	gaze-evoked nystagmus results from a normal strain on an abnormal gaze mechanism (see B above)
E	T	usually drug induced

276.
A	T	
B	F	sixth cranial nerve palsy
C	T	
D	T	
E	F	urgent treatment with thiamine (vitamin B_1) is indicated

277. A   T
     B   T   Wernicke's hemianopic pupil, classically elicited by illuminating the hemiretina which relays to the affected optic tract
     C   T
     D   T
     E   T   hemianopic 'band' optic atrophy

278. A   T   sympathetic dilating nerves are affected early in the disease
     B   T   mydriasis occurs early; later, misdirected regeneration of nerve fibres leads to miosis
     C   T   extreme miosis
     D   F   mydriasis, often with loss of light reaction, is frequently seen in cases of deep coma
     E   T

Neurology and systemic diseases

279. A   F   *contra*lateral
     B   T
     C   T
     D   T
     E   T

280. A   T   an isolated hemianopia is common
     B   T
     C   T
     D   F   a sign of *middle* cerebral artery thrombosis
     E   F   *cerebellar* ataxia occurs. Sensory ataxia indicates disease affecting the posterior columns

281. A   F
     B   T
     C   T
     D   F   indicates posterior column, rather than cerebellar, disease
     E   F   coordination, but not power, is affected

282. A   F   branch vein occlusion is frequent
     B   T
     C   F   hypopyon, posterior synechiae and secondary glaucoma are common
     D   T
     E   T   this agent has now replaced others

283. A   F
     B   T
     C   T   convulsions, hemianopia and mental retardation are due to meningeal angioma
     D   T
     E   T

284. A   T
     B   F
     C   F   low serum copper and caeruloplasmin levels
     D   F   autosomal recessive
     E   T

285. A   T
     B   T
     C   T
     D   F   this is the commonest presenting feature of *acquired* toxoplasmosis
     E   T

286. A   F   lung fibrosis is seen
     B   F
     C   F
     D   F   although hypercalcuria is found, hypercalcaemia is a feature of acute sarcoidosis
     E   F   cell-mediated immunity is impaired

287. A   F   the reverse is true
     B   F
     C   T   ischaemic optic neuropathy is seen in 90% of patients with eye involvement
     D   F   normocytic, normochromic anaemia and a very high ESR are found
     E   T   although unusual, it is a highly suggestive symptom

288. A   T
      B   T
      C   T
      D   T
      E   T   it has succeeded diethylcarbamazine

289. A   T
      B   T
      C   T
      D   T
      E   T

290. A   F   low pressure is typical
      B   T
      C   T
      D   F   lagophthalmos
      E   T

291. A   T   rubella retinopathy usually involves the macula
      B   T   cataract may be unilateral
      C   T   less common than retinopathy or cataract
      D   T
      E   F   usually patent ductus arteriosus or pulmonary
                  stenosis occur, which are acyanotic

292. A   F   inheritance is autosomal dominant, and both males
                  and females are affected
      B   T
      C   T   conduction defects on ECG
      D   T
      E   T

293. A   T
      B   T
      C   F   although these patients have a higher incidence of
                  keratoconus
      D   F   levels of IgE are elevated
      E   T

294.
A   T
B   F   intellectual development is retarded to a variable degree, despite early treatment
C   F
D   T
E   T

295.
A   T   optic atrophy and deafness
B   T
C   T   progressive renal disease, lenticonus and cataract
D   T
E   T   this comprises pigmentary retinopathy and congenital sensory deafness. It is estimated to cause 50% of all cases of combined deafness and blindness

296.
A   F   autosomal recessive
B   T
C   F
D   T
E   T   also polydactyly, hypogonadism and pigmentary retinopathy

297.
A   F
B   T
C   F   this is the myelin of the peripheral nervous system
D   T   astrocyte proliferation follows inflammation in plaques
E   T   in those patients with no history of visual loss, an abnormal VER is often found

298.
A   T   classically indicates a parieto-occipital lesion
B   F   this suggests an optic tract or lateral geniculate lesion
C   T
D   F   pupil response is normal
E   F   these occur in frontal cortex lesions. Parieto-occipital lesions cause abnormal pursuit movements

299. A T and some young adults
      B F although this is the usual indication for surgery, increased intracranial pressure and headache are commoner presenting features

      C T
      D T calcification of the tumour is typical
      E F peripheral gliosis is responsible for tumour attachment to vital structures such as the chiasm and medial walls of the hypothalamus. Atraumatic, complete removal may be very difficult

300. A T classical of hysteria
      B T
      C F this strongly suggests organic disease
      D F
      E T a seeing eye finds it difficult to avoid looking at the drum and nystagmus will be elicited

BIBLIOGRAPHY

Some of those recommended below are general texts, others are more detailed sources to which the interested reader may wish to refer. Many of the questions and answers are derived from these texts.

Basic sciences

Adler's Physiology of the Eye, 8th edn, Moses RA, Hart WM (eds), 1987, CV Mosby, St. Louis.

Clinical Anatomy of the Eye, Snell, RS, Lemp MA, 1989, Blackwell Scientific Publications, Boston.

Clinical Optics, Elkington AR, Frank HJ, 1984, Blackwell, Oxford.

Ocular Pathology: A Text and Atlas, 3rd edn, Yanoff M, Fine BS, 1989, JB Lippincott, Philadelphia.

Physiology of the Eye, 4th edn, Davson H, 1980, Churchill Livingstone, Edinburgh.

Wolff's Anatomy of the Eye and Orbit, 7th edn, Warwick R, 1976, HK Lewis, London.

Clinical ophthalmology

Atlas of Clinical Ophthalmology, Spalton DJ, Hitchings RA, Hunter PA (eds), 1984, Churchill Livingstone, Edinburgh.

Basic and Clinical Science Course, Sections 1–11, 1989–90, American Academy of Ophthalmology, San Francisco.

Clinical Ophthalmology, Duane TD (ed), 1986, Harper and Row, Philadelphia.

Clinical Ophthalmology, Miller S (ed), 1987, Wright, Bristol.

Clinical Ophthalmology: A Systematic Approach, 2nd edn, Kanski JJ, 1989, Butterworths, London.

Stallard's Eye Surgery, 7th edn, Roper-Hall MJ, 1989, Wright, London.

Neuro-ophthalmology, neurology and general medicine

The Eye in General Medicine, Rose FC (ed), 1983, Chapman and Hall, London.

Neurological Differential Diagnosis, Patten J, 1977, Harold Starke, London.

Walsh and Hoyt's Clinical Neuro-Ophthalmology, 4th edn, Miller NR (ed), 1985, Williams & Wilkins, Baltimore.